STO

ACP

DISCARDED

S0-DTQ-620

SPEECH DISORDERS

SPEECH DISORDERS

*Multisensory Techniques for Remedial Education
in Disorders of Speech, Language and
the Psycho-neural Motor System*

by

SUZANNE DE PARREL

Translated by
D. M. KEANE

✳
61687
P24s

PERGAMON PRESS
OXFORD · LONDON · EDINBURGH · NEW YORK
PARIS · FRANKFURT

Pergamon Press Ltd., Headington Hill Hall, Oxford
4 & 5 Fitzroy Square, London W. 1

Pergamon Press (Scotland) Ltd., 2 & 3 Teviot Place, Edinburgh 1

Pergamon Press Inc., 122 East 55th St., New York 22, N. Y.

Gauthier-Villars, 55 Quai des Grands-Augustins, Paris 6

Pergamon Press GmbH, Kaiserstrasse 75, Frankfurt am Main

Copyright © 1965
PERGAMON PRESS LTD.

First English edition 1965

Library of Congress Catalog Card Number 64–25230

CONTENTS

v

PART TWO

SESSIONS IN REMEDIAL EDUCATION DESIGNED FOR THE ADOLESCENT AND THE ADULT

PREFATORY NOTE

MADAME DE PARREL describes in the following pages methods for the treatment of speech disorders which, many years' experience has convinced her, are effective when used by skilled practitioners.

The phonetic content of the French spoken language corresponds sufficiently to that of the English to allow the English speaker not only the use of her methods but also of the majority of her exercises. Madame de Parrel does not, of course, prescribe exercises for the remedy of defects in articulation of sounds which are present in English but not in French, such as the unvoiced and voiced *th* sounds. For the use of English speakers, in connection with those exercises which refer to all vowels or all consonants, the vowels of English and those consonants which are additional to those of the French language are set out on pages 16 and 30.

In several respects Madame de Parrel's methods differ from those familiar to workers in similar disciplines in this country. On the other hand she enunciates principles, particularly in relation to the treatment of disorders in childhood, which will be applauded by many who see that, even in this country, these principles are by no means universally applied. Madame de Parrel strongly advocates proposals which bear reiteration: (1) early ascertainment of the disorder; (2) immediate initiation of remedial treatment; (3) acceptance of the parents and family as playing key rôles in helping the patient and, in consequence (4) the necessity for skilled counselling for parents; (5) the continuity of the therapeutic programme which, though initiated, demonstrated and supervised by the expert, must be dependent on the constant support for the remedial measures which can be given in the home.

Her work, in encouraging the increasing application of these measures, will make a fundamental contribution to successful therapy for children.

H. L. OWRID

Department of Audiology and
Education of the Deaf
University of Manchester

PREFACE

by

MAURICE AUBRY

Professor of the Faculty of Medicine in Paris

TO MAKE life worth living we need the inspiration of an ideal. The ideal which Dr. Gérard de Parrel chose as his goal and to which he devoted his conscience, his intellect and his life was a noble but ill-rewarded one: the remedial education of the deaf, and in particular of deaf children. He was one of the first to demonstrate that the child is often not completely deaf and that his residual hearing can be employed through amplification and by training. Furthermore it is unforgivable to neglect this residual auditory capacity and allow it to disappear when so often the capacity may be developed by use.

The death of Dr. de Parrel would have created an even greater gap had he not left trained pupils. The foremost of these is Madame de Parrel, his companion through life, who has continued the great work of remedial education which she regards and has often described as a sacred duty.

The methods of remedial education are not easy to acquire and they are exacting. They demand a professional integrity which is always alert and highly developed teaching qualities together with physical and moral stamina equal to every need. Madame de Parrel indeed has these qualities. I can confirm this since I have observed her untiring devotion in the work which she has carried out at my request in remedial therapy for the voice. To endow the deaf with speech and to restore it to those who have undergone laryngectomy, not to mention the improvement of less serious speech disorders, are tasks which she undertakes with the greatest skill and conscientiousness.

xi

Methods of remedial education are multiple and only too often reflect the individual nature of a handicraft. They are handed on more or less accurately from worker to worker, each of whom has his own personal method which can only be transmitted incompletely and with difficulty, like the secrets of the medieval artist–craftsmen which were handed down in succession from father to son.

Madame de Parrel's book is designed to fill this gap. She describes her method, its possibilities and drawbacks, and reveals her secrets. Her book brings home to the reader what a fund of perseverance, faith and self-denial the worker in this field must possess to pursue his task to a successful conclusion.

In her book, Madame de Parrel examines, in a manner that is clear and easy to read, the disorders connected with phonation. She describes the different forms of disability, both in the child and the adult. Every speech disorder is examined, classified and explained and the appropriate remedial education detailed. The book will be of interest to all who wish to devote their lives to the education of the deaf, for it shows what qualities of mind and body the work requires and how carefully one should deliberate before committing oneself to it. Established workers in the field of remedial education will gain new knowledge from this book and, even if their methods are not comparable, they cannot but profit from many aspects by reading it through. It will demonstrate to the doctor the importance of remedial education and will encourage him to pay attention to the voice since disorders of phonation can always be corrected if sufficient trouble is taken. Finally the patients themselves will draw from it the courage to fight against their disability. It will show them that modern medicine is at length extending aid to them so that they may regain the rightful place in society from which they have been unjustly excluded for so long.

One need not be a prophet to predict that this book will enjoy a great and well-deserved success, for the words of the author, with all her enthusiasm and her dynamic approach, are the words of faith.

INTRODUCTION

PRINCIPLES AND RESOLUTIONS

I do not practise medicine. Since 1930 I have devoted my life and the fruits of my work and efforts to the study of methods of remedial treatment for speech disorders and for multiple disabilities involving speech, language, psychomotor function and personality. I have devoted myself to the cause of those suffering from cerebro-motor paralysis and from all types of defect whether of the child or adult. Throughout this work I had before me a great example: that of Dr. Gérard de Parrel, who died, alas, in 1956. He dedicated his whole life to the noble task of the education of deaf people and children whose progress had been impeded by their affliction. He was the pioneer of remedial education in France. It was at his instigation that the Gérard de Parrel Social Centres for Remedial Education were established, where we were able between 1934 and 1946 to provide treatment and education for hundreds of patients, suffering from all types of disability.

For several years now a collective effort has been made toward the remedial education of the handicapped, but it is still incomplete and insufficient. The methodical application of multisensory techniques of remedial education produces positive results in the most complex cases. It is splendid work, interesting and effective, and in which we have complete faith. Before I die I am happy to be able to leave to those who will follow me a detailed account of the techniques of multisensory remedial education which I had the honour to create.

The techniques have beyond all doubt rendered good service and furnished evidence of their sound basis in practice. Only too often a sort of scientific snobbery has led to the creation and description in abstruse language of methods of education for use with children suffering from dysphonia and dysarthria, and with backward children; such descriptions claim to be simple but are far from being so! We propose here to furnish practical illustrations of the methods of multisensory remedial education. Those who concern themselves with this question can carry out these exercises and have them carried out in a manner at once effective and intelligible. Our aim is not to make a study of the pathology of individual cases, nor to describe the different methods of arriving at a diagnosis or a prognosis for each.

At the beginning of the century, in 1905, after numerous psychometric experiments, Binet and Simon published an intelligence scale, designed to determine the degree of retardation of children who were incapable of keeping up with their fellow-pupils owing to lack of intellectual capacity. They used a series of standardized, graduated tests (such as have continued in use in larger numbers and in improved quality), designed to establish within the shortest possible time the stage of intellectual development of the child, the so-called "mental age", and assign the child an "intelligence quotient".

The intelligence quotient is obtained by dividing the mental age by the real or chronological age.

$$IQ = \frac{MA}{CA}$$

In normal cases the quotient is equal to unity. In the case of a deficient child with a mental age of 9, and a chronological age of 12, the IQ is 9/12 = 0·75. By this criterion the idiot has an intelligence quotient of 0–0·20; the imbecile of 0·20–0·40; the mental defective of 0·40–0·85 according to the degree of retardation. An intelligence quotient of less than 0·50 indicates inability to respond to education.

During the years following the publication of the work of Binet and Simon, psychiatrists and special educationists were strongly attracted by this new method of investigation, mathematical in appearance, and offering quantitative results. Several volumes would be required simply to enumerate the studies devoted to these intelligence "tests" between 1905 and the present time. Attempts have been made, for reasons of convenience, and to save time, to establish investigational methods applicable to groups of children. The group tests established in this way have also attracted the attention of all teachers and psychiatrists.

One may think it not altogether prudent to introduce a unit of measurement into a field that is purely subjective, to claim to make a qualitative assessment, using quantitative means, and by presenting the results of a psychic examination in quantitative terms to lull the child's parents and possibly oneself as well, into a false sense of security. Besides, such tests do not attach sufficient weight to the diversity of human brains, to the complexity of their mechanism and the essentially variable conditions which govern the operation of the mental faculties and the motor centres. The aim was to tie down something essentially mobile, to photograph something possessing no clearly defined shape; it was a sign of over-confidence in the limited means at our disposal to attempt to plumb the depths of the intelligence and to trace out its exact profile.

Nevertheless, the attempt was laudable; the "test" method has provided valuable results and continues to do so. We should, however, exercise a certain scientific humility when applying it, never forgetting that "the raw material which it is designed to assess, is living matter", exposed to the sum total of the influences of its external and internal environment, to all the fears, all the contradictions and all the psychic distractions that exist.

The child who is submitted to such a test loses his bearings — may even suffer inhibition; he does not grasp why all these people, whom he has never seen before, are asking him so many questions and requiring him to make so many responses. If he feels at ease he does his best to answer, but the result is certainly below the optimum possible owing to his being taken unawares. Often his performance is below his own average; he flounders in this labyrinth, or becomes stubborn; he replies at random or not at all. Hence the serious errors which occur in the test results. Sometimes he is impeded by a hearing defect which has not been recognized or by insufficiently acute vision. He gives the impression of marked mental retardation, whereas the case is in fact one of simple scholastic retardation. Such an erroneous assessment, which we know has often been made, can give rise to regrettable faults in treatment.

Assessments, based on the tests, are moreover only one of the elements of the investigation. A precise opinion on the intellectual potential of a young subject can only be based on his being "placed under observation for a period of weeks". Such is the principle to which I, for my part, have adhered for many years and I refrain from delivering an exact prognosis of a child's accessibility to education or of his potential for recuperation on the basis of an initial examination. I have no desire to run the risk of being proved wrong by the course of events within the near or distant future.

In other words, the compilation of a dossier on a deficient child must be carried out by stages. The first stage consists of the interview with the parents during the initial examination of the child: a file started in this way ensures that nothing that emerges from the initial contact with the subject and his immediate entourage is forgotten. The second stage lasts for several weeks; it includes a series of tests arranged in chronological age groups; it is a form of secondary examination, designed to determine as far as possible the mental, motor and affective age of the child.

Professor Heuyer has written: "The child which cuts his first tooth at 6 months, walks at 12 months, produces his first phrases at 18 months and is clean at 15 months, will follow a normal course of development in relation to intelligence and character. Failure to develop normally will be due to the subsequent occurrence of a fortuitous accident of an infectious or traumatic nature".

(a) It is undesirable to diagnose as intellectual retardation that which is merely the result of a sight or hearing defect.

(b) No weight should be attached to the assertions which parents make regarding the lively intelligence of the children even in the face of patent psychic abnormality. In this respect there are no limits to the blindness of those close to the child.

(c) In regard to locomotion, the distinction must be made between "knowing how to" and "being physically capable of". As the late Dr. Pichon used to say[1]: "Knowing how to walk is only one of the elements involved in being able to walk. Knowing how to walk does not depend on motor and neuro-muscular development but on the psychological development of the individual. It is important to distinguish between motor disorders especially those affecting the gait and defects in walking of psychic origin".

(d) As regards the question of soiling the bed, i.e. sphincter muscle discipline, Pichon maintains[2] that this is a psychological and not a neurological problem.

(e) As regards the development of affective emotions, Pichon observes that it takes place in two stages: the receptive and the oblative.

Receptive Stage. At this period the only affective gratification is to receive affection, to be loved.

Oblative Stage. During this period we see added the more active pleasure of loving with all the possible sacrifices this involves. The first three occasions that involve sacrifices are: weaning, submission to sphincter discipline and the birth of a brother or a sister. Underdevelopment of the oblative function is a precursory symptom of an affective disorder, which may even go so far as "affective retardation". Where there is a total absence of affective function we are justified in being gravely apprehensive regarding the intellectual future of the child. He is likely to fall within the category of the seriously deficient. For greater simplicity let us compare the affective centre to a radio station which, if it is to function normally, must both "receive" and "transmit".

Our aim is simply to draw up, for the use of workers in the field of remedial education, a practical list of exercises to be used for the correction of the wide variety of complex disorders affecting speech and language. As far as we know no such Manual of Remedial Education exists. Many theoretical studies have been made of this problem. Their scientific value is beyond dispute but the actual work of remedial education is not described in sufficient detail.

We intend that it should be easy to apply the particular exercises appropriate to the correction of these numerous disorders, referring in each case to the notes and examples provided. A concrete example described by word of mouth is not sufficient. It is essential to have written instructions. This facilitates the work considerably. It is also our intention that all those concerned, from children's nurses to schoolteachers, including the families themselves, should have accurate information regarding disorders of speech in the baby and the child, so that these faults can be tracked down as early as possible and mitigated, or even eliminated.

Those who make remedial education their career will find here, we hope, a guide to their work. My sole desire has been to draw up a practical and detailed manual of my techniques of treatment; techniques which can be adapted to fit the multiple speech and language disorders that occur in the child, the adolescent and the adult.

My son, Louis Colle, following in my footsteps, has been responsible for the application of these principles of remedial education at Monte Carlo and in the Alpes-Maritimes. They have stood the test of more than thirty years application, and have been continually reviewed, corrected and adapted to meet developments in scientific research.

All too many methods, claiming to be based on complicated scientific studies, attempt to cure all types of defect by means of remedial education, but produce no appreciable results.

Both the psychiatrist and the oto-laryngologist have been able to achieve inspiring results in the treatment of stammering, thanks to the introduction of new drugs. It is, however, the view of the doctors themselves, that the need is for the work of medical therapy, psycho-therapy and remedial education to be combined, in order to afford the stammering patient substantial and *lasting* relief, whether he be left-handed, naturally left-handed although using the right, or right-handed.

Several workers in the field of remedial education, however, are bold enough to claim that they can mitigate this disability – or rather remove it – in a limited number of lessons. We have, alas, proved the emptiness of such claims. The foundations of our methods are energy and patience. The worker must grudge neither his efforts, nor his technical knowledge, nor his physical and mental resistance.

I consider those methods of treatment which are based on scientific conceit, practical ignorance and, to a certain extent, laziness, to be erroneous and inefficient. It is to aid in the struggle against this exploitation of misfortune and anxiety that I am listing in detail these methods of remedial education which are effective, are based on precise and pertinent observation and technical knowledge and which bear the stamp of good faith and devotion.

When a child has been subjected to the whole gamut of the famous "tests" and his mental age has been in the most approximate manner and often erroneously established, he is returned to his parents, without the slightest indication being given of what remedial treatment is required. Once the diagnosis and prognosis (whether true or false) have been made, there is no going back on it. This is the start of the stricken families' tribulation. They go from doctor to doctor while every variety of treatment is tried, including that of healers. The families carry with them their despair and bitter sorrow.

If by chance one day they come across a worker in remedial education who refuses no case but will try everything, hope returns to them. We have known cases of very seriously retarded children, who, as a result of the stimulated activation of the cerebro-motor mechanisms have gradually become conscious human beings; they have been awakened to take an almost normal place in the life of the family. They have even managed to learn to read and write.

Too many parents have their hopes disappointed. If remedial treatment is applied, the mothers may be forced to come two or three times a week with their children for sessions of twenty-five or thirty minutes without being allowed to be present during the work periods. The families are not asked to carry on with the treatment at home and no written instructions are given to them. They do not know what treatment their child has received and do not notice, even after long months of waiting, more than a vague hint of any improvement in the pathological condition of their unfortunate little one.

We take our stand firmly against this method of work. The periods of remedial education must be strictly individual and must take place in the presence of the mother or of a person capable of ensuring that the prescribed exercises are carried out at home. The process of remedial education requires the participation of the family. The child is brought once or twice a week for examination by the orthophonic specialist and the exercises are carried out twice a day at home. In centres of remedial education (which are alas extremely rare), where in-patients are accepted, educational exercises are carried out twice daily at fixed times, and the performance of the routine of daily life during the remainder of the time is itself a form of education.

I would like to wish all those who undertake this human salvage operation, the joy that I have myself experienced for the past thirty years in freeing from their fetters so many unfortunate beings, destined to live out their lives on the margin of normal humanity. I devote to them the best that is in me, the best of my work, my research, my vocation, to say nothing of the enthusiasm and spiritual zeal, without which nothing constructive can ever be attempted.

PHONATION AS ONE OF THE PRINCIPAL BODILY FUNCTIONS

The voice is the basis of human life. It is by means of the voice that man communicates with his like; in the struggle for life, the voice and articulate speech represent a powerful, irreplaceable weapon. By means of the voice, our thoughts take on audible, communicable form, patterning themselves in the amazing moulds formed by the organs of articulate expression.

But have the public authorities and all those who have to do with children and specially those concerned with education, devoted sufficient attention to the importance of the function of phonation? Do all those who have chosen a profession which brings them into constant contact with children, whether at an early or a later age, receive the type of training which will permit them to assess from all points of view the phono-articular peculiarities of those placed in their charge? Are they fitted for that indispensable task, the examination of phonation, articulation and language? It is vital to know how to listen to a child and assess its condition in regard to voice and articulation, which often keeps pace with somatic, cerebral, motor (psycho-neural) and intellectual development. Later the whole body of the teaching profession, covering all branches of instruction, from nursery classes to University courses, should receive instruction at least on the essentials of phonation, its function, its organs and how they work, its manifold forms and the disabilities to which it is liable.

From the age of 18 to 20 months onwards the human being makes systematic use of his voice. He begins to articulate and, in default of grave pathological damage, continues to do so until the day of his death. Speaking becomes as natural a process as breathing or eating, as the circulation of the blood or the secretion of the glands. At school, when he can read, he learns the importance of sight, hearing, smelling, tasting, touching and the functions corresponding to breathing, eating, the circulation of the blood and glandular secretions.

We suggest that the word phonation should take its place with the four principal functions of the human body. This would draw attention to the primordial importance of the phono-articulatory act. Children would receive at school and in college the same basic instruction on the anatomy and physiology of the vocal apparatus, its dependence on the respiratory mechanism, on the resonators, the muscles and organs of articulate expression, and the cerebromotor mechanisms which participate in the vocal function. They could also be given an introduction to phonetics and acoustics in relation to the formation of sounds, especially articulate sounds. This would be a measure of obvious wisdom and immediate value.

I hold the view that to familiarize the public, as well as the world of medicine, the teaching profession, the body of children's nurses, physiotherapists, workers in the field of education and families, with the concept of phonation, would be a good step towards realizing the only effective prophylactic measure for vocal and articulatory defects. These are far more frequent than is generally recognized and only too often they are neglected and forgotten.

To summarize, we present the following plea which, if it were heard and put into effect, would put an end to a painful situation and render humane and effective assistance to those in need; it would prove beneficial to a large number of unfortunates, reducing their numbers and improving their lot.

   i. The word "phonation" should be included among the principal functions of the human body: nutrition, respiration, circulation of the blood, glandular secretion, *phonation*.

   ii. This new nomenclature should be inserted in the text books at all levels of primary and secondary education. The study, from the anatomical and physiological points of view, of the organs, muscles and cerebro-neural mechanisms involved in the function of phonation should be adapted to different levels of teaching.

   iii. Reference should be made in these studies to phonoarticulatory defects and disorders and methods and possibilities of their cure.

PLEAS ADDRESSED TO THE MEDICAL PROFESSION

1. They should consider multisensory remedial education as an essential therapeutic measure in the treatment of disorders of audition, speech, language, physical bearing and psycho-neural co-ordination in children.

Remedial education should be combined with medical therapy as soon as the defect is recognized. In the case of the deaf child, remedial education should start at eight months.

Subjects with sub-normal hearing of all types account for an approximate 10 per cent of the total child population. Some are discovered soon enough by the parents themselves or by the family doctor. Others, if their disability is unilateral, may be regarded as lacking in mental capacity or in concentration, an error which brings heavy consequences in its train.

The deaf child has a *right* to acquire the power of speech, in the same way as the normal child. The only difference is that he must learn it by means of lip-reading and by auditory activation; it is important to begin exercises in remedial education from the age of eight months.

As regards the wide variety of deficiencies which occur in the child, we shall never cease calling on the medical profession to prescribe remedial education as an essential therapeutic measure in combination with strictly medical therapy. Let them never fob off anxious families with such criminal words as: "Wait", "The condition will clear up", "Do nothing for the time being", "It will cure itself at puberty". For all this is false. Disabilities grow worse as the child grows up, the condition is aggravated and carries a serious threat for the future. The defective child turns into a frustrated unhappy adolescent and in the end we have to deal with an adult who has become disillusioned and wretched. His young life has been spent in constant failures at successive stages in his school years; he is embittered and discouraged.

We may also consider the case of the juvenile delinquent. If he had received remedial education when he was no more than "contrary", he might have become a good citizen capable of leading an industrious and profitable existence. Such subjects require treatment at least at the age of 3 years if a history of juvenile delinquency is to be avoided.

Instruments are now available which can develop the ability of the ear to register the sound of speech and other sounds. At the age of 6 or 7 a child can take advantage of a hearing aid and as a result is no longer profoundly deaf.

The use today of the term "deaf mute" revolts the conscience. It evokes the picture of long rows of poor creatures of somnolent aspect, incapable of intercommunication except by gesture. This practice is unfortunately still current in the official Asylums for Deaf Mutes.

2. Let the expression "deaf mute", which is an inaccurate and pejorative term, be banished from the vocabularies of the medical and teaching professions.

True muteness is a symptom of aphasia, the result of an encephalopathic accident before or after birth. The deaf, however, are not mute. If those around them give them the experience of speech at the normal age for the acquisition of phonetic speech, they will be able to lip-read and speak, provided every effort is made toward the reanimation of the acoustic nerve from the age of 8 to 10 months, since very few deaf persons are totally devoid of residual hearing. "Deaf children are not invalids". They are creatures in whom one sense functions defectively. The complementary nature of the organism, however, ensures that hearing is replaced by sight. Deaf-blind subjects are equally capable of remedial education and there are some famous examples.

The deaf child is often highly intelligent. We can quote an instance of a totally deaf child who was accepted at the École des Chartes and passed out among the top students. He holds at present an important executive appointment in a large organization.

The expression DEAF MUTE should no longer be allowed currency. It is a question of human values and social respect.

3. The same principles of early treatment should be applied to dysphonic disorders in the adolescent or the adult.

Eunuchoid Disorder. If the voice of an adolescent remains unbroken beyond the normal period, he should be immediately taken to a worker in remedial education, who in a matter of moments, perhaps in a few minutes, will restore a normal male voice.

Hoarseness. The same attitude should be maintained toward the sufferer from prolonged hoarseness. Do not expect the condition to clear up by itself. After all forms of medical examination are complete, the sufferer should be sent to a worker in remedial education.

Dysphasia and Aphasia. Whether in the case of a Broca motor aphasia or a Wernicke aphasia, or where it is simply a case of a more or less marked dysphasia, remedial education of the patient is essential as soon as possible after the accident to the cerebral cortex which has caused the speech and language disability.

4. *Laryngectomy Patients.* For the acquisition of the voice per oesophagum the same principles apply. It is a good plan for the patient to be sent to the architect of the vox per oesophagum BEFORE the laryngectomy is carried out (since this is a question of "education" and not "re-education"). The patient for whom laryngectomy is proposed is thus accustomed to the use to be made of eructation. The brutal shock which is normally occasioned by the production of the vox per oesophagum is avoided. One thus obtains in advance, a psychic compliance in the act of producing belched sounds. After the ordeal of the operation the patient remains sometimes for several weeks in a state of asthenic debility before his level of comprehension allows practical results to be achieved. It is therefore important, where material circumstances permit, that the patient should be brought to the worker in remedial education two or three weeks before the operation. In any case, as soon as possible after the wound has healed.

5. Regular medical examinations should be instituted in nursery schools, where children are accepted from the age of 3 onwards, to ascertain the child's state of health in regard to physical and motor phonetic functions. Such examinations should be carried out by a pediatrician, an ophthalmologist, an oto-laryngologist who specializes in disorders of phonation, and a psychologist.

If the smallest disability is recognized the child should be sent at once to the worker in remedial education. In this way, by the time he reaches school age, the child will have been permanently freed of his fetters.

REMEDIAL EDUCATION

Remedial education is a method of functional adaptation, related to therapeutic physiology and psycho-pedagogy. It aims at the awakening, correction or replacement of the living mechanisms which control human activity in all its various forms. It has the following immediate objectives:

1. To bring into operation organs which, as a result of arrested development (pre- or post-natal), have never functioned.

2. To readapt those functions which have lost their normal activity.

3. To replace functions which, as a result of accident or illness, have become atrophied.

WORKERS IN REMEDIAL EDUCATION

I shall not discuss in this article the qualifications and diplomas needed by those carrying out the profession of remedial education in speech by multisensory methods. They are already well-known: matriculation, degrees, diplomas in phonetics and psychology, training in music, long term training with qualified orthophonic specialists.

I give first priority to those physical and moral qualities without which no one can claim to be an effective worker in the field of remedial education. I would not advise those without physical strength or without strength of mind to commit themselves to this career. Remedial education is a sacred duty. It should not be undertaken except by those with exceptional qualities and gifts. In a task of this kind the pursuit of financial gain has no place. Long and careful reflection is vital before committing oneself, since it is a hard, tiring, arduous and financially unrewarding profession.

This said, I remain convinced that remedial education is the most wonderful and the most socially rewarding profession.

Physical and Moral Qualities

The physical qualities required are: stamina to meet any demand; good health; attractive physical appearance; good sight; perfect hearing; well-developed larynx (strong voice, faultless articulation); absence of local or foreign accent; deep, easy breathing; strong heart; muscular suppleness.

The moral qualities needed are: inexhaustible imagination; self-denial; selflessness, energy and the power to captivate; the vocation for teaching; the gift of placing oneself permanently at the disposal of others; generosity; lack of egoism; an infectious gaiety; intuition; psychological acuteness; intelligence; goodness; detachment; absolute love for one's profession combined with an impassioned optimism; constant desire to encourage and inspire complete confidence in the sufferer, to impart energy and hope and unflagging morale; the possession of an equable but lively disposition; the ability to ignore jealousy, over-susceptibility and malice; and never to expect real gratitude. One must have the desire to save and to mitigate or cure suffering without expecting any reward except the consciousness of duty done. Rigorous self control is necessary: the ability to restrain or control the impulses of one's own personality, to dominate them and never to allow oneself to give way to anger. In a word to place all one's knowledge, patience, all one's moral, physical, intellectual and spiritual forces at the disposal of those who are entrusted to the talents of the remedial teacher.

One must have the ability to make a diagnosis and to adapt the educational treatment in a manner appropriate to each case. Remedial education, especially that for phonetic and psycho-neural motor disorders must be related to the individual. There are as many cases as there are individuals and the treatment must be specially adapted to each one according to his inclinations, his possibilities, his intellectual potential, his sensitivity or nervous excitability. Remedial education cannot be "standardized" without losing its efficacy.

It is the imagination of the remedial teacher which spontaneously works out the exercises, adapting them to the daily needs of the sufferer. It is seldom that one finds a patient exactly as one left him. Every hour, every day, there are changes in his mentality, his energy, his will. One must know how to take advantage of the good days and very often of bad moods, to get to know the patient and apply appropriate treatment. Only in this way will one be useful and able to bring help to the patient.

CATEGORIES OF DEFECTS TO WHICH THE MULTISENSORY METHODS OF REMEDIAL EDUCATION ARE APPLICABLE

Defects of speech and language	Dysphonias (children, adolescents, adults) Dyslalias (children, adolescents, adults) Aphasic patients (children, adults) Laryngectomy patients (vox per oesophagum)
Intellectual and psychological disorders	Those who are educable. Those who are partially or completely defective. Backward pupils. Mongoloid types. Psychopathic subjects (defects of personality).
Sensory deficiencies	Completely deaf subjects. Partially deaf subjects. Hard of hearing children.
Defects of psycho-neural motor co-ordination	Those who are subject to psychomotor instability and fatigue. Patients with slow psychic or motor reaction. Stammerers. Stutterers. Mumblers. Simple hypotonics. Normal faults. Patients with disturbed rhythm. Adult stammerers.

Patients suffering from myopia, organic motor defects, impotence, paralysis due to muscular atrophy, various forms of myopathy and polyneuritis are not included in the above categories. Such patients require the type of remedial treatment provided in functional recuperation centres, fitted out with the necessary equipment for physiotherapy, mechanical therapy, short wave and infra-red treatment, radio-therapy, light baths and radiation treatment. This is not within the scope of our activities.

PART ONE

Remedial Education Sessions Suitable for Children

I SHALL only concern myself with correct speech and the remedial education of the psycho-neural motor function, where the governing factor is the energy, the dynamic imagination and the competence of the remedial teacher.

The exercises, which I shall describe during the course of the sessions of remedial education, cannot, of course, be carried out during a single period, but the prescribed sequence should nevertheless be followed. The order is not to be changed.

It is the task of the remedial teacher to decide on the number of exercises appropriate to a particular working session. The patient must be watched carefully, to catch the first signs of physical or mental fatigue and distract him where necessary. Never end a session with a refusal or a setback. A pupil should leave his teacher, filled with satisfaction and confidence, and the desire to see him again. The sessions should be made attractive, interesting, absorbing, not only for the child, but for the mother also.

On undertaking a case requiring remedial treatment, the worker should ask the person who brings the child to provide a bound notebook. In this book he will write down the exercises which he has just carried out during the session and which are to be repeated twice daily at home. This will constitute in effect the complete account of the treatment and will remain in the possession of the family, so that from time to time, they will be able to continue the prescribed exercises for purposes of further training even after the disorder has been alleviated.

I shall not mention in this short work remedial techniques involving the use of visual and plastic materials. Their qualities both visual and tactile as well as their value as a means of intellectual and scholastic remedial education need no further demonstration. They are known throughout the world and are constantly being developed. The Decrolys and Montessoris and their pupils are

3

continually producing new and effective equipment. I give due credit to these benefactors of the backward child.

Here I am concerned only with the creation and improvement of speech and language; with the stimulation of cerebral activity by means of psycho-neural co-ordination, that is to say: the training of the cerebro-motor mechanisms by means of the simultaneous execution of dissociated movements of the parts of the body, such execution being linked with thought and its immediate form of expression: the spoken word.

CHAPTER I

DYSPHONIA – RHINOLALIA
(NASAL SPEECH)

POSITIVE AND NEGATIVE NASALITY –
HOARSENESS – GUTTURAL SPEECH

There are two forms of rhinolalia or nasal speech.

1. *"Open" rhinolalia or hyperrhinolalia:* an alteration in the timbre of the voice owing to the predominance of the nasal resonator, where there is permanent communication between the buccal and nasal cavities as a result of perforation of the hard palate, paralysis of the velum or a hare lip.

The vocal timbre is distorted, as are all the consonants apart from: *m, n, ng.*

The palatal and velary inadequacy results not only in nasal loss and a nasal twang in the speech, but also in compensatory facial grimaces and faulty positioning of the point of the tongue, when articulating the dentals *t, d, l,* or the sibilants *s, z.*

2. *"Closed" rhinolalia or "hyporhinolalia":* This condition corresponds to obstruction of the nasal cavity by the growth of tissue or by any other mechanical obstacle. If the obstacle is located in the anterior section of the nasal fossae, this results in negative nasality; if it is located at the rear, the subject cannot nasalize vowels and there is distortion of the consonants *m, n, ng.*

A simple method of distinguishing the rhinolalias is as follows: make the subject pronounce *ah* and *ee* several times, alternately closing and opening the nostrils. In the case of "open" rhinolalia the tonal pronunciation of the two vowels changes, whereas for "closed" rhinolalia they remain the same.

Finally there are forms of nasal speech which result from velary paresis or paralysis of cerebro-motor origin. In this latter case the dysphonia is only one of the symptoms of a general syndrome, of which the prognosis is poor.

The remedial methods applicable to such psycho-cerebral motor deficiencies will be dealt with later on. It is in any case of prime importance to attempt to reduce first of all the level of dysphonia. Those whose nasal pronunciation is due to a hare lip are, as a rule, intelligent and the results of treatment are decisive — treatment should be given as soon as possible after surgical intervention, as early as the healing process allows, since the surgical rectification requires to be followed as soon as possible by phonetic remedial education, in order on the one hand to gain correct articulation of the distorted sounds and on the other to accustom the ear to the sounds now correctly reproduced.

No sufferer from nasal speech can pronounce the guttural *r* nor the fricative consonants *zh* (as in plea*s*ure) and *sh* (as in *sh*e). The subject appears to be speaking with the mouth open. The voice is hoarse and muffled.

AN EXAMPLE OF A SESSION IN REMEDIAL EDUCATION

To induce suppleness and to give motor training to the articulatory organs:

(a) Lower the maxilla (lower jaw) as far as possible in a single movement.

(b) Close the mouth in a single movement, pressing the jaws together very hard.
Duration: half a second per operation (repeated 30 times).

(c) Move the maxilla forward sharply, opening the mouth at the same time with the lower teeth in front of the upper incisors.

(d) Move the maxilla to the rear, while opening the mouth wide (30 times).

(e) Open the mouth completely.

(f) Put the tongue right out.

(g) Close the mouth again.

The exercise is carried out in 3 time, which is beaten with both hands stretched well out (sitting position):

1.	2.	3.
Strike the knees	Open the arms wide in a single movement	Strike the shoulders

These movements must be carried out very rhythmically, the one position being succeeded immediately by the next without any intermediate pause, in time with the movements of the maxilla and the tongue (30 times).

(h) Clear the throat violently several times, opening the lips and stretching the cheeks to the maximum at the same time. It is difficult to make the subject carry out this exercise energetically at the first attempt. It should be persevered with, since it is of decisive importance in order to bring the whole glosso-pharyngeal apparatus into operation (30 times per session and to be prescribed 100 times per day at least).

(i) Press the lips tightly together (so that the mucous surface is invisible. While in this position make a sound with the mouth closed for the space of half a second, then jerk out the three syllables pa! ba! ma! These syllables should be clapped on the child's hand. The teacher can compare the sharp sound to the explosion of a small bomb, which amuses the pupil (40 times). Make a sound with the mouth closed, followed by the same a sound with the mouth wide open (40 times), the sounds being produced afresh each time.

(j) Inflate the cheeks like a balloon, then deflate them, hollowing the cheeks (20 times).

(k) Push the lips well forward, shouting the vowel oo (as in moon). Open the lips as wide as possible, shouting ee (as in seen) (50 times in the morning and in the evening).

(l) When the vowels are being pronounced correctly, with the proper timbre, they should be articulated with each consonant* in turn, in a loud voice:

* See page 30.

boo–bee, koo–kee, doo–dee, foo–fee, goo–gee, choo–chee, loo–lee, moo–mee, noo–nee, poo–pee, roo–ree, soo–see, too–tee, voo–vee, xoo–xee (ksoo–ksee), yoo–yee, zoo–zee.

These syllables should be worked over from the first to the seventeenth and back from the seventeenth to the first in rhythmic time with the following movements, to be performed with energy: strike the breast with both hands: extend the arms sharply (the whole process to be repeated 20 times).

(m) The tip of the tongue should be smacked against the front part of the hard palate (25 times).

(n) Work on the sharp articulation of the following in a loud voice:

> *ka! Gan!*   from *ka* to *rran* and
> *kan! Goua!*   then return from *rran* to *ka*
> *rra! rran!*

the vibration of the *r* to be stressed. (The exercise should be done 60 times per day if possible).

(o) When an improvement in the dysphonia is noted, at the end of some ten sessions, the young dysphonic subject should be made to articulate a series of syllables which he finds difficult.

EXAMPLES: *galleon, grant, whistle, corvette, clap, crackle, dragoon, ectoplasm, trousers, scream, garden, cruiser, crinoline* (each word to be worked over at least 20 times).

(p) Conjugate the following verbs as shown below:—
I grind corn. (1st, 2nd and 3rd persons singular and plural).
I crack the branch.
I crunch sugar lumps.
I attend a crowded class.

(q) If the syllables *nyo* — as in *onion*, and *nya* — as in *banyan* are incorrectly articulated, which occurs frequently with nasal defective speech, they should be practised directly in speech work, e.g. *canyon, minion, onion, banyan, lanyard, companion, pannier, union.*

(r) The same attention should be paid to the syllables *mia* and *pia*, practising them directly in the words, *piano*, *opiate*, *miaow*, *amiable*, *Pierrot*, *impious*, etc.

(s) It is also of value to make the child count (if he is able) from 1 to 100 and 100 to 1. Particular attention should be paid to ensuring the correct pronunciation of 20, 70 and 90, which are often difficult for nasal subjects.

(t) This sequence should be carried out in exact 4-time, which is beaten with arms extended (stiff as rods) in the sitting position:

1.	2.	3.	4.
Strike the thighs	Cross the hands on the breast	Extend the arms wide	Strike the shoulders

If the child is incapable of counting easily from 1 to 100 and 100 to 1, the following technique should be adopted. Count from 1 to 10 and 10 to 1 several times, then from 10 to 20 and 20 to 10. Then learn the numbers 1 to 20 by heart and proceed by progressive stages of 10 up to 100.

The treatment for a negative nasality follows the same practical methods as for nasal speech. Negative nasality normally originates in a slight paresis of the velum, accompanied by auditory adaptation to the distorted sounds. In the treatment of negative nasality, as for all phono-logical therapy, the auditory habits must receive remedial education at the same time as the speech defect.

Remedial session for twice daily performance

(a) Exercises of the maxilla and clearing of the throat. Stretching of the naso-labial groove. *(Basic exercises should never be omitted)*.

(b) An exercise involving the production of sounds with closed mouth.

(c) An exercise for the correction of distorted sounds.

(d) An exercise involving various words which present difficulty to the subject with a nasal speech defect.

(e) Exercises involving appropriate phrases or the conjugation of verbs.

GUTTURAL SPEECH — HOARSENESS

These two almost similar types of dysphonia are characterized by the localization of the vocal resonance in the lower pharynx. If such troubles result from some form of irritation or a scar, they are to be treated by the medical specialist. In the child, however, they are generally functional — resulting from overtaxing of the larynx or errors in the voice production.

Many children misuse their speech organs from a very early age by excessive crying, a phenomenon often nervous in origin. Babies who "howl" day and night for months, possess a marked hoarseness from the moment they acquire the power of emitting the first spoken sounds. This disability becomes aggravated later and we have very often found guttural speech and hoarseness in children of 3 to 4 years.

Another danger, and a very serious one, makes itself felt when the young pupils are made to sing at the start of their school life. School teachers and teachers of singing, having received no training in relation to phonation and language, have no knowledge of the vocal possibilities of the children. Moreover it is not the custom for a pulmonary and laryngeal examination to be carried out by a medical specialist concerned with voice and speech production before the children are allowed to take part in choral singing. Like adults, children (both boys and girls) have low, medium and high voices. They are made to sing, irrespective of their own capabilities, in whatever range happens to suit the requirements of the musical work; this results in the straining or maltreatment of the vocal respiration, the vocal muscles and the whole laryngeal apparatus.

I entirely agree that singing is of practical use from more than one point of view. Children's singing should, however, be governed by their powers of vocal delivery, their muscular capacity, the soundness of their auditory apparatus and their respiratory control. In default of this children gradually begin to develop defects of delivery, muscular fatigue and, in consequence, hoarseness. They speak and sing with a constant huskiness, and the shouts they produce during the recreation period are hardly designed to improve this condition.

When children suffering from such forms of dysphonia are brought to me, I start by imposing, as far as possible, a regime of vocal abstinence.

I request their teachers to excuse them all vocal singing.

I then set in train remedial treatment on the following lines:

1. Full lowering of the maxilla, together with closing of the mouth, slowly but without hesitation (40 times per day).

2. Several respiratory and spirometric exercises (twice daily); exercises involving the nose and the mouth.

3. The vowel *ay* — as in *bay* — to be pronounced with sharpness, but lightly, briefly and in tune (guide-note: E natural 4th on the piano or any other musical instrument). Ten times successively for one operation *ay!ay!ay!ay!ay!ay!ay!ay!ay!ay!*

The subject will not achieve this at the first attempt since the vocal cords cannot meet this requirement. This is of no importance. Even if the voice is husky, the vowel *ay* should be attacked sharply, opening the mouth wide and stretching the labial joints (angles of the lips) as far as possible.

This series of ten sharp vowels should be repeated ten times per day, using discretion as to the lightness and briefness of the sound. During each session of remedial education conducted by the teacher 20 vowels may be attempted in this way, but families should be instructed to carry out the prescribed exercises (in series of 10) ten times.

4. *60 times* per day, with the lips pressed together and the mouth closed, attack the sounds in the high register. This will be practically impossible at first, but after a few days the exercise can be performed 80, 100, 110, 120 times, and even greater numbers of sounds should be achieved progressively with the mouth closed as a daily exercise.

The child should experience internal vibratory sensations behind the upper incisor block.

5. When the vowel *ay* has been achieved in an incisive manner on E (4th), the vowel *ee* should be attacked in the same way on the

note F (4th) natural or F sharp, or if possible G. The notes should be attacked lightly and briefly, without causing fatigue and above all, without forcing, then

6. proceed from *ay* and *ee* to the vowels *a* — as in *pat* — and *wa*, attacking them in the order *ay, ee, a, wa* (20 times).

7. Then articulate in the normal voice, linking the syllables: *ba, bwa, bee, boo, bo, bay*, all six syllables to be pronounced during the same breath (20 times).

8. Each of the following phrases should then be articulated twenty times in a clear voice with precise articulation:

I must articulate properly when I speak (conjugate the verb for all persons, singular and plural).
My voice is much clearer now.
I must not shout and tire my voice.

Articulation must be carefully watched during this exercise.

If it is carried out with energy and correctness, it will do much to relieve the speech organs and muscles.

9. When at the end of a period varying from one month to three, the young pupil has acquired a clear, normal voice, the parents and teachers should be recommended not to let him sing for at least a year and then only if there has been no recurrence of hoarseness.

CHAPTER II

DYSLALIA–DYSARTHRIA

ALL defects of articulation in its proper sense fall under this heading.

1. Defective articulation of certain speech sounds (consonants, vowels, syllables).
2. Inability to articulate the consonants: *b, p, y, k, r, l, d, t, f, v, s, z.*
3. Incorrect pronunciation of certain vowels: *e* — as in *the, ay* — as in *day, oo* — as in *too, wa.*
4. Confusion of guttural and dental consonants and substitution of the one for the other: *ga* for *da, ka* for *ta, se* or *she* for *fe, ze* or *zhe* for *ve.*
   EXAMPLES: *mekro* for *metro, tow* for *cow, krain* for *train, sut* for *shut, grag* for *drag, bajar* for *bazaar.*

A fantastic variety of such substitutions are found. The most common examples are those given above, but the examination of any large population of speech defectives can reveal surprising examples of incorrect articulation which have never previously been encountered.

In certain cases there is a physical basis for such types of incorrect speech. The most common reasons are gaps or deformations of the dental arches, an excessively acute arching of the palate, incorrectly positioned or anomalous incisor teeth, maxillary atresia, lower jaw out of alignment, anomalous development of the incisor block, the upper lip and the tongue.

If the lower jaw is out of alignment (glossoptosis) the incisor rows no longer meet. As a result the flow of air is distorted, dispersed and deviates for its proper course. The consonant *s* loses its sibilant character because the tongue comes up against an impediment at the point where the air leaves through the gap between the teeth: the *s* becomes softened to *sh*.

Maxillary atresia, resulting in a reduction of the transversal diameter of the bone, is likely to give rise to articulation defects since it restricts mobility of the tongue, causes faulty positioning of the pre-molar and molar teeth, produces interdental gaps and reduces the volume of the buccal resonating cavity. The whole range of speech defects can thus be observed to occur as a result of this anomalous condition which is so frequent, but so frequently goes unrecognized for want of a systematic examination of the child during the pre-school period. The artificial transverse dilation of an arch which is too narrow, if it is carried out in time, will allow the teeth to move of their own accord into their proper positions and achieve a correct functional balance. The family doctor and the dental surgeon are in duty bound to co-operate in such measures to protect the health of the child; it is not only a question of protecting the child against irritating speech imperfections of a maxillo-dental origin, but of putting its respiration and mastication processes on a sound foundation, safeguarding its facial appearance from the aesthetic point of view and fostering its bodily and psychic development.

The most ordinary forms of dysarthria, brought to remedial teachers for treatment, are "sigmatisms", or lisps.

The underlying causes of sigmatism may be physical, malformation of the lower maxilla, malformation of the roots of the teeth, slightly, very slightly defective hearing, whereby the high-pitched vibrations of the voiced and unvoiced sibilant dental consonants *ze* and *se* are alone affected.

This slight hearing defect, to which we refer, is perhaps only the defective adaptation of the auditory mechanism to the incorrect pronunciation of the sibilant dentals. The child gets used from a very young age to hearing its own incorrect articulation. His ears come to accept the sound of this distortion. The reason why phonetic therapy takes so long to carry out is the need for auditory adaptation to be effected. This is true of all forms of re-education, affecting pronunciation and language, since the faulty articulation gives rise to faulty auditory adaptation. Lisping can in some cases be *acquired by mimicry, where the father, mother or some member of the family has an impediment in speech.*

REMEDIAL EXERCISES
FOR SIGMATISM (LISPING)

1. As for all remedial education sessions for phonetic disorders, begin with the *basic* exercises. *Never omit them:*

   (a) Lower and raise sharply the maxilla *thirty times night and morning* (each movement to take half a second) followed by energetic projection of the maxilla in a *lateral direction* with the mouth wide open (30 times morning and evening).

   (b) Projection of the maxilla in the *forward* and *rear* direction with the mouth wide *open* (30 times morning and evening).

These exercises have the advantage of imparting suppleness and tone to the muscles and the articulatory organs, provided they are carried out with energy, precision and abruptly. They also force the subject to carry out rhythmic and precise movements, thus training his motor control. They provide an excellent cerebral exercise, preparing the child for psycho-neural co-ordination exercises.

2. Clear the throat violently at the base of the throat 80 times (the intention being to render supple the organs of the mouth, larynx, pharynx and the base of the tongue).

3. Run the *tip* of the tongue in a rotary motion over the *outer* edges of the gums (behind the lips), keeping the mouth firmly closed, then blow out the upper and lower lips again in a rotary direction (exercise for the tip of the tongue). Carry out six times in succession. Stop and begin again 20 times per day. Since the lisping subject introduces the tip of his tongue between the incisors during articulation, the tip of the tongue must be trained to avoid this incorrect movement.

4. Clench the teeth firmly. Open the lips as wide as possible. Retaining this position, whistle lightly, but with *as pure a tone as possible*, behind the teeth, making sure that the tongue remains behind the incisors. *Sssssssss* (the noise made by a small saw) *200 times per day.*

5. When the consonant *sssss* is sounded correctly and purely, *and only then*, add to it, with a pause between, the vowel *a: sssss ... a.* Take particular care not to pronounce *sa* as a single syllable *in the first instance*, since the child will slip back into the original fault and again introduce the tip of the tongue between the incisors. Auditory adaptation takes quite a long time to achieve.

If the child is properly taught and works hard and attentively each day, the articulation should be satisfactory at the end of a *fortnight*.

6. If the child begins to get the pronunciation of the *sa* right instinctively, he should be made to practise the *s* with all the vowels:* the consonants depend in fact on the vowels which precede and follow them. Practise the following vowels: *a, ay* — as in *day*, *ee, o* — as in *pot, oo* — as in *moon, oa* — as in *boat, wa* — as in *swam, er* — as in *heard, wi* — as in *swim*, always stressing the vowels *er* and *a* (20 times per day). *Practise loudly:* do not mumble or whisper.

7. Practise the voiced sibilant *z* in exactly the same way. Compare the sound of the *zzzz*, made with the teeth clenched and the lips open, with the noise made by a mosquito in flight.

---

* The vowels of English are set out below and reference may be made to this list when the text refers to exercises involving all the vowels.

Short vowels	Long vowels	Diphthongs
i as in *bit*	*ee* as in *feet*	*ay* as in *day*
e[1] as in *bet*	*ar* as in *father*	*ou* as in *go*
e[2] as in *apart*	*or* as in *bought*	*ai* as in *my*
a as in *bat*	*oo* as in *moon*	*ow* as in *now*
o as in *pot*	*er* as in *heard*	*oi* as in *boy*
u[1] as in *put*		*ia* as in *here*
u[2] as in *but*		*ea* as in *there*
		oa as in *boat*
		ua as in *poor*

8. When the improvement in articulation has become automatic, practise the same consonants in the weak position. Consonants can in effect occupy three positions in the word:

EXAMPLE: the consonant *s*

(a) Strong position, in front of the vowel: *salute, satin.*
(b) Weak position, after the vowel: *race, pass, glass.*
(c) Inter-vowel position: between two vowels in the word: *assent, ascend, massage.*

9. It must not be forgotten that for subjects with defective articulation, the consonant is more difficult to pronounce in the weak than in the strong position. The following syllables should, therefore, be practised correctly 20 times per day: *bass–mass–nass–pass–rass–sass–tass–vass–yass–zass.*

10. Practise in the same way: *baz–kaz–faz–daz* etc.
It is also of value to practise the same exercises with the vowels: *a ay ee o oo oa wa er wi.* Examples: *bayz–kayz* etc.

11. When the lisp impediment has been improved, groups of syllables such as the following should be pronounced:

> *gra–za–sta–*
> *spay–ray–assay–*
> *stee–zee–assee–*
> *apso–sto–asso*

12. Make up phrases on the lines of the following — or easier phrases if the child is too young to articulate these.

EXAMPLES: make a phrase with the word *sea* or repeat ten times — *the sea is blue,* a phrase with the word *pears* such as — *I saw some sweet pears,* a phrase with *lesson, basin, Jason, massive, immense, azalea, Mississippi, swat, asthma, design, Lazarus, question.* The field is wide and the remedial teacher must always keep his imagination alert.

13. In the case of the unvoiced and voiced consonant combinations *ks, gz* which are seldom well articulated, it is of value to

practise under two heads: *ks* unvoiced as in *excess* and *gz* voiced as in *examine*. The two forms should be practised, using the syllables: *kessa, kessay, kessee, kesso, kesswa*, articulated rapidly to accustom the child to the simultaneity of the syllables in *ksse*. Then the same exercise using: *guza, guzay, guzee*, etc. followed by the words *access, examine, extraordinary, taxi, axe, box, excess, excite, exaggerate*, etc.

These words are also practised for the voiced and unvoiced forms in order to achieve the automatic elimination of errors: the child should get used to stressing the gutturals *k* or *gue* in the body of the words.

EXAMPLES: *aksses takssi ek stra ordinary bok ss ek sses eg za gerate eg za min* etc. Any method of this sort, which achieves success *(suk–sses)* is good. The result is the important thing. Success can always be achieved if sufficient trouble is taken. The curing of sigmatism is a long process; we should never deceive ourselves about this. It sometimes happens that a malformation of the lower jaw gives rise to a prognathous (protruding) effect in the upper. In such cases surgical intervention by the dentist is essential.

Slurred pronunciation is, in addition to sigmatism, one of the imperfections in speech most commonly met with. Slurring is the incorrect articulation of the fricative consonants, both voiced and unvoiced *je she*.

Sometimes these phonetic sounds are completely lacking. In other cases the poor articulation is complicated by a lateral positioning of the tongue in the interior of the mouth and even by a twisting of the lips at the moment the phonetic sound is attempted. The sound produced by this attempt is unpleasant, while the accompanying grimace shocks the observer. Substitution of the fricative sound for the pure sibilants often occurs and vice versa. The remedial education can be greatly helped by the use of a mirror, if the child is capable of appreciating the movements which give rise to this faulty articulation.

1. The first exercises to be carried out are the basic exercises already referred to.* The throat clearance exercises must not be omitted.

2. Then, if the muscles of the lips and cheeks are twisting at all, practise with a strong voice the production of:

oo, forcing the lips and cheeks forward

ee, opening the lips as wide as possible.

3. Make the subject articulate very loudly *boo bee*, preparing the way by forming the phonetic sound *b* with the lips pressed tightly together, so that they burst apart (30 times morning and evening).

4. Then instruct the child to clench tightly the rows of incisor teeth, pouting out the lips as much as possible: in this position, blow out a loud *shsh* behind the teeth, in imitation of the puffing of a steam train; the tongue should of course be held behind the teeth (at least 100 times per day).

5. Carry out the same exercises as for sigmatism. Articulate the consonant *shsh* separately from the vowels, then, after the articulation and auditory adaptation of the child have become automatic, together with the vowels. In order to keep the young pupil amused, small pieces of paper may be placed on the table. As the child puffs out the *sh*, he attempts from a distance to move the heaps of paper; the teeth are of course pressed together.

6. Work on the *zhe* in the same way. *Zhe* is in general an easier sound to reproduce than the unvoiced sound.

7. The same consonants are then practised in the weak position: *ash, cash,* etc. and in phrases with *bash, cash, harsh, garage, blancmange, grange, beige, moustache, hush, branch, flange, punch, mesh,* etc. If examination reveals or gives reason to suppose the impediment in the speech is accompanied by defective hearing, retarded hearing (a slowing down of the speed of auditory perception), defective hearing in certain ranges or by the restriction of auditory sensitivity to high-frequencies only, the family should be advised to consult an oto-laryngologist. The doctor will arrange,

* See page 9.

if he feels it necessary, for an audiogram to be taken of the child's auditory fields, since any disparity in bilateral auditory sensitivity may result in articulation defects.

During the process of remedial education of a child who is able to read, avoid exercises involving reading aloud. An essential element of the remedial exercises is that they should stimulate cerebral activity in the child. The imagination is now evoked by reading and the child, owing to the distraction offered by the text, neglects the effort to articulate correctly and starts once more to mispronounce the phonetic sounds which have already been practised. Devices to depress or in any way guide the tongue should not be used. The child must produce by means of his own effort and will, the proper sounds. He listens, builds up and achieves the sound, modelling himself on the examples given by his teacher, while his brain, under the constant stimulation, increases continually his reserves of will-power and rhythmic activity.

A tape recorder is a first-class aid in all treatment for the remedial education of speech and articulation. After a few working sessions, the child becomes extremely sensitive to the sound of his own voice. The use of a tape recorder is recommended in order to establish the progress that has been made. It is desirable that a recording, however brief, should be made during the first examination. This method of assessing the progress made provides a conclusive criterion for the child himself and his family. The remedial teacher will himself find this means of checking progress advantageous.

CHAPTER III

DEFECTS IN THE PRONUNCIATION OF CONSONANTS AND VOWELS

K AND *G*

These are frequent

A child of normal auditory and intellectual capacity acquires speech between fifteen and eighteen months and two years. Often the articulation of certain words remains inaudible because certain consonants are distorted or omitted, e.g. the unvoiced and voiced gutturals, *ka–ga*. In such cases remedial exercises should be started as soon as the deficiency is discovered. All the basic exercises and throat clearings should be carried out immediately. The use of a tongue depressor is indicated. The tongue is thus held against the bottom of the mouth and the child can only articulate by using a combination of the base of the tongue and the soft palate.

1. In this position, articulate with maximum resonance in the voice: *a* sharply (60 times).
2. Then clear the throat and sound the vowel *a* loudly.
3. Now practise *ka–ga*.
4. When these are obtained correctly the pupil should articulate them in combination with the vowels: *a–ay–ee–o–oo* (as in *goon*), *oa* (as in *goat*), *wa–wee–er*.
5. Then the same thing in the weak position.
6. Articulate words in which these gutturals are located in the three positions given on page 17.

EXAMPLES: *garden, bag, agriculture, cultivation, become, back, maggot, gutter, fog, poker, cup* etc.

Complete phrases should of course be made up with each of these words. This is where — I repeat — the remedial teacher must draw on an inexhaustible imagination in adapting the exercises to the progress made by the pupil, making them attractive, amusing and instructive.

All this cannot be learnt in a day. One must be careful to refrain from indicating to parents a probable date when a positive result can be expected from the treatment. In some cases achievement comes very quickly, in others the delay must be regarded simply as grounds for redoubling one's efforts.

OMISSION OF THE CONSONANT L

In cases where the consonant *l* is observed to be lacking (we have deliberately refrained from using such terms as lambdacism, rotacism etc. which are not generally understood and have no practical value), the child who fails to articulate the *l* should be given, at the start of the process of remedial education, exercises to practise the use of the three sectors of the tongue: base, middle and tip.

1. Clearing of the throat deep down, carried out shortly and sharply.

2. An exercise consisting of rapid vibrations of the tip of the tongue against the outer part of the upper and lower lips. Imitation of the movements of the tongue, such as are made to amuse babies: produce first the syllables *ba* or *pa*, if they exist, followed immediately by the lingual vibrations

> *ba llllllllll* vibrations of the tip of the tongue
> *pa llllllllll* vibrations of the tip of the tongue

This movement is very hard to carry out to start with. The pupil will only be able to move the tongue out for a single movement, but the whole exercise will be rapidly grasped and learnt, if the teacher pursues it with energy (100 times per day at home).

3. An exercise of the semi-consonant (palatalized consonant) *ya*, designed to raise the back of the tongue toward the bony palate. Initially attempts should be made to obtain articulation of the syllables *ya, you, yan, yon*, which should then be incorporated in words.

EXAMPLES: *million, billion, onion.*

4. An exercise for the tongue: maxilla as low as possible; touch with the point of the tongue:

> –the *front* part of the *upper* incisor block
> –the *front* part of the *lower* incisor block
> –the *right*-hand corner of the lips (outside)
> –the *left*-hand corner of the lips (outside)

(this exercise to be repeated 40 times per day).

5. Put out the tongue forcefully, make it pointed, then in a slow relaxing movement, flatten it out. This exercise is not easy to start with, but is especially effective in mobilizing the transverse muscles of the tongue (20 times per day).

6. If the child is slow to grasp this, make him touch with the tip of his tongue a tongue-depressor, placed to the front of the mouth, and at the same time pronounce *la.* Whilst the tongue depressor is licked lightly the sound will be rapidly achieved.

7. Once the phonetic sound *l* has been mastered, it should be practised in the inter-vowel and weak positions in all the normal syllables and using all the vowels, until it becomes automatic. The following are examples of words for practice: *galleon, loom, omelette, ball, control, lesson, vessel, Polly, flower, molar, allusion, total, miserable, table,* etc.

Form verbs to conjugate or short phrases, incorporating all the above words.

ABSENCE OF THE PLOSIVE DENTAL CONSONANTS *T, D,* AND THE NASALS *N* AND *NYA*

In such cases, after finishing the basic exercises, the upper and lower rows of teeth should be brought together noisily. The child should then be made to bite several times (at least 20 times) on a tongue-depressor, which is rapidly withdrawn at each attempt to bite (this exercise is particularly valuable for children who find difficulty in masticating their food); it should be made clear to him that the sounds *ta* and *da* are pronounced with the teeth directly opposite each other, in order to give the consonant the necessary force, without the tip of the tongue being inserted between; he should be made to appreciate the difference by the energetic articulation of *la*, then immediately afterwards *ta*, the unvoiced sound *t* is generally mastered much quicker than the voiced consonant *d*. To achieve this latter sound as in the case of all the voiced sounds, the child must be shown how the vocal cords vibrate in the articulation of all the voiced consonants. This can easily be achieved by placing the hand on the thyroid cartilage (Adam's apple).

When the dentals have been mastered carry on in the same way as for the other consonants by means of work on the syllables, followed by the incorporation in words and phrases of these consonants.

EXAMPLES: *Tea is an invigorating drink, the task is interesting, turn down the tabs, the chocolate drops are delicious, the teacher is strict*, etc.

It is of value to articulate these words in 3 or 4 time, beating the time with both hands, one syllable per beat.

Time: $\frac{1}{4}$ second per beat.

Articulation of the nasals *na* and *nya* should be treated in exactly the same way as the plosive dentals (voiced and unvoiced) which we have just dealt with.

The child who cannot produce these sounds must above all be taught the habit of bringing the rows of teeth exactly opposite each other, in order to do so. It follows that the consonant *n* is acquired by means of the same exercise as for the dentals. First of all the child's nose is closed with the hand so as to accustom him to the nasal sound. With children who find it difficult to assimilate the *ye* sound in the nasal *nya*, after mastering the *n*, the sound *nya* should be split up into its components *ni* .... *a*, linking the sounds together. If necessary the hand should be slid across the table in time with the exercise. The child pronounces the *nee* at the start of the movement, continuing the sound throughout and adds the vowel at the end. The resulting sound is: *neeeeeeeeeea*. The movement of the hands helps to form the sound. Follow the same procedure with the remaining sounds.

EXAMPLES: *nee .... a   nee .... ay   nee .... o*
nee .... oo   nee .... oa (as in *boat*)
nee .... er (as in *heard*)

Follow up with the words: *minion, banyan, onion, canyon, lanyard, union, companion*, etc.,
Finally phrases should be formed in order to make the pronunciation of these phonetic sounds automatic.

ABSENCE OF THE
FRICATIVE CONSONANTS *F, V*

This articulation deficiency is one of the most rapid to remedy.

1. Remedial education should be begun in this and all other cases with the basic exercises, those designed to practise the movements of the maxilla, the tongue, the lips and the cheeks, and throat-clearance at the base of the throat.

2. Make the child bite on his lower lip. It is as well for the teacher to use his hand initially to maintain this dento-labial position. The child should then be made to blow very hard behind the lip which is being held. The teacher himself blows on the child's hand in the same way.

3. When the movement of puffing out the lower lip can be carried out correctly and easily, the usual vowels are added with a break between the consonant and the vowel *fff–a–fff–ay–ff–o–ff–oo–ff–oa*.

4. Practise the same thing with the consonant *v*, first separately and then in syllables with the vowels.

5. Allow your imagination free rein to produce suitable words or practise the consonants associated with the *l*.

EXAMPLES: *infant, affair, fool, fresh, fantasy, fluff, safe, grave, mauve, love, fray, flower, vase, fraternal, float, flutter, vine.*

Conjugate the verbs:
I offer my mother some flowers (all persons, singular and plural),

I eat fried bread, you eat, etc., *I dive in the pool, you dive,* etc.,
I feel very well, etc.,
Repeat each exercise ten times.

ABSENCE OF THE BI-LABIAL PLOSIVES *P* AND *B*, AND OF THE BI-LABIAL NASAL *M*

Cases where the voiced and unvoiced labials *b, p,* are lacking are rather rare. In general even deaf children acquire them through instinctive lip-reading. We have, however, occasionally found this phonetic deficiency in certain children with speech impediments or aphasia.

It is easy to cure. We recommend the adoption of the following techniques to eradicate this impediment.

1. Practise the basic exercises.

2. Using his hand, the teacher should press the child's lips one against the other, so that he experiences the physical sensation of contact. With certain disorders the patient is lacking in awareness of his own person, or body image.

When contact has thus been established, make this consonant explode against the back of the teacher's hand and then against the child's hand. Children are in general very quick to grasp this little game. Points to be stressed are the firm closing of the lips and the energetic movement to expel the sounds from the mouth. The child must not be allowed to inflate his cheeks to produce these labial sounds. This is quite wrong.

3. When the articulation of the sounds *pe....a* and *be....a* has been achieved several times, the usual syllables should be practised so as to articulate the labials in the three positions.
EXAMPLES: *pa, pay, pee, po, poo, pwa* (30 times, followed by the same syllables in association with *b*).

4. Then treat in the same way the syllables: *ap, ayp, ab, ayb,* etc. (30 times); and finally *apa, aypa, eepa,* etc. *aba, ayba, eeba,* etc. practising with all the vowels (20 times).

5. Finally practise large numbers of words, involving the articulation of these two consonants:

barrow, baton, parry, tumble, rabble, carp, loop, tablet, apartment, etc. (20 times per day).

Phrases should be constructed containing each of the above words.

THE BI-LABIAL NASAL *M*

This bi-labial sometimes takes a long time to master.

1. Start as for *p* and *b* but with a long pressure on the lips, then make the subject produce a sound with the mouth closed and open his lips gently, with the lips pressed first against the teacher's hand, then against the subject's own hand: *mmmmmmmmmmmm mmmmmmmmmmmmmmm* (60 times).

2. Have the subject articulate the *mmmmmmmmmmmm* sound again, pressing lightly on the nose at the same time in order to bring home the nasal element in the consonant. Practise this sound with the usual vowels, but detached from them: *a–ay–ee–o–oo*; then practise the normal combined syllables: *ma–may–moo* etc; finally the same consonant in the weak and inter-vowel position: *am aym eem om um oom anm onm inm* and *ama ayma eema oma uma* etc.

Practise also in the words:

marine, Mary, motor, millet, man, Tom, hammer, come, amusement, amity, omniscient, human, imam, etc. Suitable words are easy to think of.

3. Practise articulation of the phrases with each of these words.

INCORRECT VOCAL TIMBRE

Many subjects with speech defects render the following vowels unrecognizable owing to the incorrect timbre of the voice: *oa oo ee ay wa i ai oi* are barely differentiated. As a result words and language become very hard to make out. A child will for example say *stumble* for *stubble, fraze* for *freeze,* and *my car* for *my cow.* Apart from cases of defective hearing, this is due to an infantile aphasia, resulting from a difficult or critical childbirth or from some form of encephalopathy.

Specialists in speech disorders and remedial education should be aware of the classification of the vowels, so as to be able to appreciate properly the distortions of the timbre of the voice which occur in the speech and language of many speech defectives.

The phonetic sounds are grouped in accordance with their articulatory characteristics, their range and type of resonance (see p. 29).

TECHNIQUES TO REMEDY DEFICIENT OR DISTORTED VOCAL TIMBRE

Vowel deficiences, involving the small and large rear resonators, affect principally the *oo*, *o*, *ee* and *ay* sounds.

The phonetic sound *a* is almost invariably mastered even in serious cases of lingual or velary paresis.

It is sufficient to carry out breathing exercises on the lines of the artificial respiration administered to a drowning man, sounding a long *a* during expiration. Unless the child is extremely deaf, he will rapidly imitate the sound. Once the *a* has been mastered, the starting point has been passed and the child will acquire the remaining vowels by mimicry.

The teacher opens his lips, as if to smile, and produces, as loudly as he can, a high-pitched *ee*. It is a good idea to start with the vowel *a*, sounded with the mouth wide open, transferring with a sharp movement to the *ee* position with undiminished resonance. Quite a long time is often required to master this sound, but if the exercises are practised enough at home the sound will soon be acquired.

oo is generally obtained with the lips pushed well forward. The child notices that the *oo* sound involves the almost complete closing of the lips and imitates this position quickly enough. Work on this sound can be ended with the game of *cuckoo*, in which the face is covered and abruptly uncovered.

Vowels requiring slight rear resonance with some examples of vowels of this type.	short a	apt, attract, pat, battery.
	short u	Venus, fuss, porous, bus, luck.
	long u (oo)	tool, fool, cool, loop.
	medium u	cook, look, took.
	short o	top, lot, hottentot, compliment, stop.
	medium o (or)	talk, cord, fork, cork.
Vowels requiring considerable rear resonance with some examples of vowels of this type.	er	pert (this sound also corresponds to other written vowels, e.g. first, work, curt, etc.).
	short e	pet, check, melt, lent, bed.
	long e(ee)	meet, feel, congeal, conceive.
	short i	rip, flick, quick, bid, pick.
Vowels requiring unique type of resonance (Pharynx, Nose and Pharynx, Mouth) and examples of words corresponding to each type of vowel.	long a(ay)	pate, lake, place, fade.
	long i(ai)	strike, right, tripe, side.
	medium a(ar)	car, park, shark, start, harsh.
	long o(oa)	cope, elope, motion, stole.
	ow	foul, cowl, howl, towel, shower, bower.
Vowels in which nasal resonance predominates and examples of words with each type of vowel.	ion	million, canyon, onion.
	ian	banyan.

The vowel *o* is easily obtained by making a round mouth. Draw a circle on paper, let the child follow it round with his finger, and in the same way feel the round shape formed by the mouth. It is unusual not to acquire this sound by the end of the third period. As soon as a vowel has been mastered, it should of course be practised in conjunction with all the consonants in the three positions, in the following order*: *b–k–d–f–g–j–ch–l–m–n–p–r–s–t–v–x(ks)–y–z.*

I do not agree with methods of remedial education which involve the use of the tongue-depressor, and the use of manual techniques to produce phonetic sounds in the child with dyslalia or aphasia.

It is both quicker and more logical that cerebral, auditory and articulatory learning should take place simultaneously and spontaneously. Our aim is to achieve this, and without the help of pictures. This requires great energy and a dynamic approach from the teacher, but the results achieved will be in proportion to the effort made.

Discrimination between the *wee* and *ouee* sounds is sometimes difficult. Some subjects with speech impediments pronounce the word *wheat* as *oueet* and the adjective *sweet* as *soueet*. So *soueet* is a very common expression among speech defectives. In such case this sound should be practised in such a way that the *w* is articulated first, immediately followed by the *ee*, in order to establish the automatic auditory association of these two phonetic sounds.

EXAMPLES: *wh…eat, sw…eet*, etc.

In the same way, if the sound *ooi* is distorted, separate it into *oo–ee* and the sound will soon be achieved.

The vowel *ay* sometimes takes a long time to acquire. Starting from the position associated with the phonetic sound *ee*, transform the sound into *ay*. In this case auditory adaptation is the

* Additional English consonants are those represented by italicised letters in the following words: *ch*ild, *j*est, si*ng*, *th*ick, *th*is, *h*at. The sound represented by the letter *x* above is strictly a consonant continuation.

road to achievement. For the deaf, of course, there is a different approach as will be seen later. Words can be made to help in the acquisition of this sound.

EXAMPLE: *away* — throwing an object down.
This phonetic sound is often mastered very quickly.

The single resonance vowels are obtained by the same methods as have been applied to those involving the small and large rear resonators; in this case there is no question of altering the timbre of the voice, which adjusts itself almost automatically. The difference between *hash* and *harsh* is simply a question of auditory discrimination and it is easy to get this over to a subject with sound hearing. The only phonetic sound which may be incorrectly learnt is the *wa*.

It is a good thing to practise this syllable split in two *oo–a:*

EXAMPLES: *oo–addle — waddle, koo–ack — quack.*

CHAPTER IV

DEFECTS OF MENTAL
AND PSYCHIC ORIGIN

TOTAL OR PARTIAL DEFECTIVES,
RETARDED OR MALADJUSTED PUPILS,
MONGOLOID TYPES,
DEFECTS OF PERSONALITY
AND CHARACTER

I cannot stress too often that defective children are rarely defective in one sphere only. We are faced with a combination of defects. I have already given techniques designed to cure dysphonias, dyslalias and speech impediments and I would like to stress again the prime importance that attaches to the re-education of the function of speech, wherever this is possible; speech is the keystone in communication between the child and those who surround him. *Top priority* must in my view be given to the creation, improvement, correction and adaptation of the speech function in the child.

Educable defectives are sometimes classified as mental defectives. They have been subjected to a series of tests providing standardized and often incorrect criteria. This elastic classification of mental defectives covers those children who have been unable to master the elements of writing, reading or arithmetic at the normal age, apart from those children for whom this failure is due to non-attendance at nursery or primary school, a long-standing illness or a serious auditory or visual deficiency.

The average defective child in this group has been a late developer, has not learnt to talk at all, or only badly, using distorted or inverted words and a minimal vocabulary. During the second

32

half of their early childhood, from two to six years, such children have been unable to learn by example from what goes on around them, to assimilate the commonplace background of everyday life and learn from imitating, assimilating what they see. Their faces are not alert, they play little and without life, and everything they attempt is marked by slowness and clumsiness.

Intellectual deficiency, if authenticated, is always accompanied by a certain level of motor deficiency. The clumsiness of the hand has its root in the brain. The slowness of the one entails slowness in the other. If such children are not given attention when it is urgent that they should have it, i.e. before they complete their third year, then the scene is set for an unending history of failure, disappointment and agonizing grief. Everything is tried, advice is sought here, there and everywhere. No advice can have any value unless it sets the child on the road to remedial education, *the only means* of effecting a cure.

No words of mine can be strong enough condemnation of the ignorance or indifference of those who give voice to those words, which are so frequently heard: "Wait a bit — the condition will clear up — it will cure itself". It is *criminal* to deceive parents in this way and to thrust into darkness a little human being who could perhaps have been cured. Only too often we have observed the dramatic and disastrous results of an attitude of this sort.

When a child is brought to me, who is mute as a result of retarded development, I observe it with devoted attention and carry out various small tests. In the course of observation of this type, I have often been able to catch a sudden furtive glance, most revealing in regard to the possibilities of awakening the understanding of the child. It lasts only for a fraction of a second. Once this revelation has been vouchsafed, throw hesitation to the winds and set to work on the treatment. How often in my career as a worker in remedial education have I been privileged to receive this sudden illumination with its promise of a hopeful outcome, and how often has that hope borne fruit!

There are also unfortunately incurable cases, where the child drags itself around on the floor with continual oscillation of the head or constantly rocks from side to side or backwards and forwards, dribbles, soils itself, gives no sign of recognizing either persons or things, is unable to chew or devours food voraciously. Under such circumstances it is better for the child to be removed from the family circle.

There are also other cases in which the poor child presents an almost normal physical appearance and even follows the treatment to a certain extent, but he emits a series of sharp cries, is subject to violent fits during which he throws himself against the walls, tears his clothes, hurls toys and other objects about the room, bites, grasps, pinches and plays with his excreta. Such cases which we have had the misfortune to meet on occasion, fall within the field of the psychiatrist. These are the symptoms of schizophrenia and must be treated in proper institutions. There is no alternative, since these unfortunate little ones — boys or girls — are a source of great disturbance in the home. They are actively harmful and constitute a danger to their unfortunate parents, brothers and sisters. Their immediate entourage should be protected from their involuntary misdoings.

EPILEPTICS

In addition to these two categories in which there are impassable obstacles to remedial education there is yet another type of deficiency which does not fall within the groups more frequently encountered. For children within this category we naturally attempt to carry out remedial education according to the severity of the symptoms but this is done only in individual sessions separate from any other group of children. I am speaking of the epileptic or epileptoid subject.

The diagnosis is strikingly obvious if one is faced with the dramatic spectacle of a real epileptic fit or with a detailed description of the symptoms, given by the parents. I do not intend to consider the medical aspect of such cases, but merely to deal with them from the point of view of the remedial teacher and the speech specialist.

In some cases the child displays no obvious symptoms and is not subject to fits. The convulsions are replaced simply by automatic movements, sometimes unobtrusive, which are carried out during work or play. For the space of a few seconds the child is quite unaware of his surroundings. He sees things without perceiving them, there is a lacuna in his psychic activity; then order is restored without the poor little one being aware of this fleeting lack of consciousness. Such is the case of the epileptoid. In more serious cases the child may wander; he escapes, walks on at random, with a complete lack of responsibility for his actions. This is called "epileptic absence". But the compulsive actions of the epileptic may on occasion constitute a danger: violence, theft, the breaking of glass are all committed in a state of complete unconsciousness. It is as well, however, to remember that compulsive epileptics may also be conscious of their actions and *remember them*.

The epileptic child is often capable of responding to remedial education and may sometimes be of normal intelligence. The obstacle to the child's recovery of his phonetic and psycho-motor function and his academic rehabilitation is his abnormal psychic state. Personality defects of varying levels of intensity are frequently met, irascibility, wildness, opposition to authority and an impetuous disposition. Such children are subject to unreasoning explosive attacks of anger and brutality, which occur against a background of irritability and over-accentuated emotional development. They are fighters, a fact which renders them dangerous to their companions during play. It is therefore desirable that they should be kept in their own family circle.

The behaviour, articulation and language disorders to which these children are subject and their failure to comply with school discipline are amenable to our methods of phonetic and psycho-neural remedial education. It will therefore be of value to refer back to the remedial exercises which we have described in relation to the treatment of those patients, whether completely or partially defective, who respond to remedial education. As regards their illness, such epileptoid or epileptic children should be placed in the hands of a medical specialist who is well qualified to prescribe treatment.

The majority of cases are fortunately not so serious. Those who are educable, even if they display a serious degree of retardation, deserve all that the devotion, knowledge, patience and imagination of their teachers can bring about.

Let me quote the case of a young boy, for whom the most influential medical advice could do nothing because, at the age of almost nine, he presented a picture of an almost total phonetic nullity. All motor and psychic tests which were applied proved negative. He was brought to me in this state by his mother, a fine woman driven frantic by a mother's love and by her determination at all costs to awaken the flame of consciousness in her child's mind.

There was only one favourable factor: a relatively high standard of cleanliness. The child was not dribbling and, although drawn and haggard, recognized his father and mother. A victim of total aphasia, the child could produce no single phonetic sound, vowel or consonant, exhibited a complete indifference to life around him and an ambivalent motor function.

I began multisensory remedial therapy out of a spirit of admiring pity for the mother. There was no question in this case of attempting phonetic mimicry; at the outset, I simply carried out the psycho-neural motor co-ordination movements, in order to stimulate the cerebro-motor neural mechanisms.

This was the procedure followed:

1. I made the child carry out the following movements, standing upright (at the beginning the movements had to be guided by hand):

    —raise the arms
    —stretch the arms out horizontally
    —lower them to the sides, shouting *one*,
       two, *three*.

Carry out ten times during each remedial session.

2. Lying down (on back) on the floor

    Raise the legs, shouting *Legs*
    Lower the legs, shouting *Legs*

Raise the arms, shouting *Arms*
Lower the arms, shouting *Arms*

(The teacher should go down on all fours for this exercise).

At the start the child let himself have the exercises performed on him without any personal reaction.

3. Standing up, carry out rhythmic strokes on pieces of white paper spread around on the ground. The child's hand must be stretched well out.

4. In the sitting position, make the child strike the table with alternate hands (outstretched) observing a close rhythm; this exercise to be carried out, it must be understood, with the teacher holding the child's hands and shouting very loudly:

Right   Left

At the end of two weeks, the mother, in transports of delight, informed me that the child was carrying out these movements alone.

5. I then prescribed some more complicated movements: in the upright position, raise the arms, touch the toes, return to the upright position, simultaneously raising the arms, then touch the ground with energy on the right and on the left. All these movements are carried out to a rhythmic count of *one, two, three, four, five,* to inculcate into the child a sense of rhythm and to develop the cerebro-motor control and accustom him to the feel of the ground.

6. At this stage attempt to make the child walk in time, with some light object on his head. He should move six paces forward, six paces back; with some help this will become automatic. Practise this at least 15 times in each period, increasing the weight and dimensions of the object carried on the head.

At the end of a month of this treatment, which was devoted solely to psycho-neural motor co-ordination, I was able, still stressing the combination of movement, cerebral effort and achievement, to obtain the phonetic consonants *pa* and *ba*, which was a victory in itself and marked the beginning of directed cerebral effort. Gradually I obtained from the child the other consonants.

The gutturals presented no great difficulty, whereas the sibilants, and fricatives were not so easy to master.

7. The child, from his state of complete unconsciousness, was slowly coming to a realization of himself, as I made him indicate with his hands: the eyes, the ears, the nose, the mouth, the shoulders, etc., pronouncing the name of the appropriate organ, with whatever degree of success could be achieved at first.

8. This pupil is now eleven and a half years old. He is following the curriculum of school lessons with a private teacher (after sixteen months of remedial treatment, he was able to familiarize himself with letters and syllables, since, like many defectives, his memory was sound).

He is now starting to read, first by copying, then in response to dictation; he can count and carry out simply little calculations. He learns poems, spells forwards and backwards simple words like: sun, mat, red, milk etc. He can, for instance, name the tools necessary for the carpenter's craft. He can dress and feed himself without help and can lay and clear the table for meals. His case represents a cure within his family circle and it is now hoped to train him for a profession. This is one of the successes achieved by the method of multisensory remedial therapy in the space of two and a half years. Thus the restoration of a child to the family circle with the ultimate prospect of learning and following a profession must be set against the bleak alternative of depriving the mother of child and child of mother.

It goes without saying that the remedial treatment is continued, where required, in order to consolidate and exploit the results so far achieved.

MONGOLOID DEFECTIVES

The child is born a mongol, he does not become so. The root cause of mongolism has not, moreover, been traced with certainty. Before discussing it, I should like to define this disorder and describe the conditions applicable to it.

Mongolism is a congenital dystrophic complex, which manifests itself in the form of mental defect, functional disorder and bodily malformation, recalling notably the characteristics of the mongol race, from which the name is derived.

This state was first described by Langdon Down in 1866. Since then many child specialists from many different countries have devoted close attention to this particular form of mental and physical deficiency. From among the hundreds of contributions made to the subject in France, let us select the monograph by Pehu in the issue of *Medicine* for August 1936, Dr. Maurice Bourgouin's doctorate thesis, published in 1938, and from the same year a memorandum by Professor Turpin, whose discussion of the subject is particularly discerning.

The Mongol Type

The name "mongol" was given because children suffering from this form of deficiency have the narrow lidded eyes of the true Mongolian type. In fact, however, they differ greatly from these latter and could therefore better be described as mongoloid types. They do not even have the protruding cheekbones, which are so typical a feature of the Asiatics. They differ moreover from the true Mongolian type in stature, cranial shape and even in facial profile.

Let us examine them in greater detail. First of all the eyes. The distance between the inner corners of the two eyes is less than normal. The palpebral slits are not horizontal, but sloped outwards and upwards. This disorientation is a characteristic feature. In many cases there is an anatomical basis for this: the epicanthus forms a sort of third eyelid and covers the inner corner of the eye. The epicanthus has become separated from the upper lid and enfolded in the skin of the cheek, tracing a line in a concave direction, downwards and outwards. Conjunctivitis and dacryocystitis are common symptoms. The lobes of the ears are badly shaped, asymmetrical and often discontinuously formed. The skin of the cheeks is red and on occasion scaly; the hair is dry, straight, fairly plentiful, but the eyebrows tend to be underdeveloped.

A point of detail: both the forehead and the back of the head fall steeply, another contrasting feature of the true Mongolian type. The skull is at once micro and brachycephalic. The tongue is large, grooved and loose-skinned; it often hangs out and the child dribbles. The hands are short, thick-set, and soft like bats. The thumb is short and the index finger slightly curved, with the concave side facing the third finger. The thumb and index finger are of approximately the same length.

Mongoloid types are small; they are reduced scale models of children. Their skins are pale and often given to oedema. They suffer in winter from stubborn and deep-rooted chilblains; very often they exhibit dermatic infections of the impetigo type in the region of the face, which cannot be got rid of. A characteristic feature of the mongoloid type is the incredible degree of looseness in their speech articulations; they would make perfect recruits as indiarubber men or clowns. Their favourite position is the Buddha posture or, put more prosaically, sitting cross-legged like tailors. The hypotonic state is their kingdom. Of all subjects, who are amenable to remedial therapy, these are the most friendly, the best-mannered and the most amusing; they know how to earn our love.

This does not alter the fact that they are retarded over the whole range of human activity; they cut their teeth late, learn to walk late, grow slowly, learn to speak late. They chew badly and swallow badly. From the point of view of mental capacity, the deficiency is generalized, but varying in degree. Complete idiocy is the exception. Some have a fairly alert memory and considerable talent for mimicry; we shall see to what use these advantages can be put, in spite of the fact that their attention is constantly wandering.

Their voices are hoarse, their utterance explosive. Prior to remedial education, the child can only repeat the last syllable of each word. He is an aphasia subject and almost always a chronic stammerer.

For the remedial education of such children, as indeed of all children, the participation of the mother or a person prepared to devote herself to the hearing of the exercises, is essential. The exercises prescribed should be carried out at least three time a day at fixed times. The brain, like other organs of the body, works better if it works regularly.

The age of the mother is a factor of primary importance in the case of a mongol child, especially where the family history abounds in cases of disability. Where the mother is still young, pathological or hereditary factors are often found to be operating, leading to premature aging. In this case the chronological age no longer presents a valid picture owing to the existence of a morbid condition.

The following table has been drawn up, relating to the age of the mothers and covering forty cases:

Four mothers aged from forty-five to fifty years
Four mothers aged from forty to forty-five years
Eleven mothers aged from thirty-five to forty years
Eleven mothers aged from thirty to thirty-five years
Six mothers aged from twenty-five to thirty years
Four mothers aged from twenty to twenty-five years.

Although mongolism is a special form of deficiency, it is extremely variable in its consequences. In the majority of cases the mongoloid type, who still possesses a sufficient basis for psychomotor function, is capable of readaptation. He is able to blend into the family background and may even manage to make himself useful. He may be able to make himself understood and understand what is said to him.

Sometimes the mongoloid must be classed with the totally ineducable cases, but this is the exception. In such cases, tragic as they are, there is no alternative to a psychiatric institution.

The vitally important thing is to begin remedial treatment *as soon as possible*. The mongoloid child does not sit up before twelve or thirteen months. Up to that time it cannot even hold its head straight. It topples over backwards. Even in the most advanced cases there is no indication of a future ability to stand upright and walk before twenty months.

Thirty months is the latest date at which a decision should be taken on the introduction of remedial treatment.

It should be stressed once again that mongoloid children react in radically different ways to the advances of the remedial teacher.

Some show rage, opposition or simply clumsiness; there are aphasics, often sufferers from myopia, those who continually sway to and fro or who are constantly moving round, or those in the grip of a sub-total apathy, who merely stutter. The general run of mongoloid types, however, are gay, amusing, fond of joking and playing, dirty, emotional and given to wheedling.

REMEDIAL TREATMENT

There can be no question of a "standard" method of remedial education for mongoloid children, any more than there can be for any other form of psycho-motor deficiency. The teacher must study his pupil, look for points of access to him and adapt the method to the child. The naturally emotional disposition of the average mongoloid child assists the teacher to obtain the love of his pupil, to interest, amuse and distract him and make him laugh.

If the child lets his tongue hang down (the tongue of the mongoloid being thick, loose-skinned, longitudinally grooved and with projecting papillae fungiformes) it becomes an impediment in the mouth; the first need is for the basic exercises to be performed, i.e. exercises for the maxilla, lips, and tongue, and violent clearing of the throat.

If the mongol is of a contrary disposition, he can as a rule be brought to an obedient frame of mind by means of games or orders which are easy to carry out, such as have been described in relation to the educable defective.

At the start of the remedial treatment, it is the psychoneural co-ordination exercises that produce the most tangible results. The pupil is first of all made to carry out (in the upright and lying positions) the exercises described in connection with general defectives who are amenable to remedial education. Subsequently these exercises are carried out on orders from the teacher.

The education of the mongloid child is the most delicate, complex operation of all; it is not a virtuoso performance, which earns admiration, but an exhausting and laborious task, ill-rewarded and often unrecognized. The smallest positive result is a victory dearly won at the price of sustained effort, requiring not only method and perseverance, but also faith. The teacher will also have to bear with the child's mother, father and immediate family, who continually watch, comment and assess his progress, passing from joy to despair in constantly fluctuating moods.

After the mongol child has learnt to obey, it will be of value to have him carry out the following exercises:

1. Walk forwards and backwards, carrying an object on the head, in order to awaken the sense of balance in the child (10 minutes per day in two sessions).

2. Exercises designed to develop cerebral rhythm.

Was it not Dr. Leon Foucault who advocated the acquisition of an *internal rhythm*, created by the child itself, as opposed to the rhythm imposed by the beat of a metronome or stimulated by some sort of musical means?

The child, seated at a table, places his hands face downward on sheets of white paper, held down with drawing pins. The teacher draws round the outline of each hand.

The child then places his hands in time on the figures drawn out in this way, first on the right, then on the left (lifting the other hand). He will require assistance to carry out these movements initially. The teacher counts *1 2 3 4* or says *right left* as the case may be, maintaining perfect rhythm and tempo (30 times morning and evening).

3. (a) The child is taught to join hands with the fingers intertwined in the attitude of supplication, a movement which is not easy to achieve at the start of the treatment, followed by

(b) a sharp movement to fling the arms wide open and bring the hands together again (30 times in succession morning and evening, pronouncing aloud at the appropriate time: *Together! Apart!*)

4. Make the child crawl on all fours with the legs stretched well out (forwards and backwards), saying the names of fourlegged animals at the same time. Examples: *dog, cat, sheep, rabbit* (10 times).

5. Immobility exercises, if the mongoloid is given to continual movements.

6. Upright position — hands on the hips — legs apart: lean forward with energy and throw oneself back very forcefully; lean over to the right without moving the legs, then to the left, pronouncing loudly:

> forward!   back!
> right!   left!
> (20 times morning and evening)

If the mongol child is left-handed, the teacher should pretend not to notice, but watch carefully and bear the point in mind during the performance of the comprehensive exercises.

Defectives of this type often experience considerable difficulty in throwing back the head to look at the ceiling ... Many victims of other forms of psychic deficiency are the same ... They must therefore be trained to carry out this movement energetically. The underlying cause is a lack of balance, a tendency toward giddiness and a fear of falling.

7. Immediately after the foregoing exercise, draw the child's attention to whatever is placed to his right, to his left, behind him or in front of him.

8. Rhythm and orientation exercise. A slate is placed in front of the child, on which are written in different coloured crayons:

> | | High | |
> |---|---|---|
> | Left | Middle | Right |
> | | Low | |

The child sits with hands crossed, looking at the slate, raises his arms and points in the direction shown in the appropriate colour.

Stretch the arms up in the air, saying: *up*. Then lower them, leaning forward and saying: *down*. Stretch the arms to the *right*, saying: *right*. Then stretch them to the *left*, saying: *left*. Finally clap the hands energetically, as if applauding and say: *in the middle* (20 times morning and evening).

9. Some more advanced mongoloids, who are able to read and write, suffer from a sort of phonophobia (fear of speaking aloud). In such case the following exercises should be performed in the upright position with the legs apart and the hands joined. Raise the arms in the outstretched position, separate the hands and place them on the feet, then stretch the arms above the head, bringing the hands sharply together, then lowering them together to touch the feet. All movements of course to be carried out in measured time.

These movements should be accompanied by the vowels *wa! a!* pronounced as loudly as possible (50 times a day).

Alternately with the above vowels, practise *grran grra*, vibrating the *r* with maximum force.

10. Hands on the hips: stretch one leg forward, bend the knee and again stretch; beat time on the floor, articulating in a resonant voice, one syllable per beat, "I must speak much louder" (30 times per day).

11. Insist on the child getting used to speaking aloud and articulating with energy in everyday life. Pretend not to hear when he speaks too softly.

12. In the course of study, attempt to interest the mongoloid in various manual crafts, making him state the tools used in each, again with appropriate rhythmic movements carried out in time with the words.

EXAMPLE: carpentry.

Enumerate: nails, plane, pincers, pliers, screwdriver, gimlet; imitate exactly the motions of hitting a nail on the head, saying at the same time: *I hammer the nail into the plank with a hammer;* then go through the motions of planing, saying: *I plane the oak with the plane* and the movement of screwing with a screw-driver, saying: *I screw the lock on to the door.*

There is a free field for the exercise of the imagination by remedial teachers: I must point out that mongoloid patients can develop favourably, thanks to present-day medical treatment. The best of them are capable of making themselves useful in some simple operation, e.g. kneading the dough, handling a plane (I know of one case highly skilled in rudimentary carpentry) working as wood-cutter, gardener (such large-scale operations as digging and raking), packing, in fact in all manual tasks not requiring the exercise of initiative. They are trainable and even conscientious and can manage up to a point to avoid being a burden on their families. This in itself is a notable achievement, since defectives of this type have long been the despair of their parents and of those who, on the death of their parents, have become responsible for them. It has long been accepted that mongoloid children die young. This is, however, no longer an exact statement, since medical therapy has been able to extend their expectation of life considerably.

I shall not concern myself in this work with the remedial education of such defectives by means of pictures or the wide variety of educative games, lotto and its successors, which provide excellent preparation for learning to read, write and count. I intended merely to give a few practical exercises of the comprehensive remedial therapy type, which might be of assistance to these unfortunate creatures, by stimulating their cerebral mechanisms into activity. Such preparatory work may then be followed under conditions of greater alertness and lucidity by more profitable forms of instruction. In view of the absence of thought processes, frequently found amongst mongols, any stimulus to understanding and intellectual activity is a valuable aid.

THE PERVERSE CHILD

Praiseworthy attempts have been made on the part of both public organizations and private institutions to deal with the problem of juvenile delinquency. All possible means have been tried in order to effect the recovery of and restore to their place in social life minors who have committed serious crimes, ranging from theft to murder by way of every conceivable form of revolt and brutality.

Previously "juvenile delinquency" was a symptom which manifested itself between puberty and maturity. Now the average age is lower; the notorious "blousons noirs" (black shirts) or the "new wave" claim members of eleven and twelve years old! This is the danger threatening the family and the social system in general. The increase in the birth-rate, the decline in the influence of the school owing to the large numbers of pupils, accompanied by the reduction in the number of available teachers, the material difficulties of life, the television, the cinema, the inability of parents to deal with the education of their children, broken homes, divorces and the evil seed sown by certain amoral publications have all combined to achieve the corruption of the young and directed their attention toward regrettable ends. "Bad examples", beckon them on every hand. Only such organizations as the Boy Scouts, Girl Guides and work camps are beneficial. They instil the team spirit, the sense of healthy comradeship, they encourage the young to get out in the open and take part in sporting activities where all must work together for the good of the team.

I shall never cease to study what is in my view the best countermeasure to the social scourge that "juvenile delinquency" has become. I mean a method of re-education, which is comprehensive, sensible and dynamic in its approach, to deal with the *perverse child*. *"The delinquent is a perverse child who has grown up". "The perverse child is a delinquent in embryo."*

The perversity of children can be classed under two heads: inherent perversity and acquired perversity. The former emerges from the very earliest years and extends its activities further and further afield as the subject approaches adolescence; if his inclinations are allowed free play, the perverse child advances from fault to fault, from misdeed to misdeed, on his way to theft and ... crime.

An acquired character defect may be the result of an affective disorder; a child, who has been an only child up to the age of three may be gravely upset by the arrival of a brother or a sister. Accustomed to being the sole object of the affection of his parents, he is at first astonished, then disappointed, to see another baby enjoying the same prerogatives. A jealousy complex emerges and with it a group of mainly painful feelings, capable of making the child naughty, cruel, violent or sulky.

Action must be taken at once. At this stage the perverse feeling is present least frequently and least seriously, since for the greater part of the time the visits of other children amuse and distract him and give him a sense of the importance of his person and his rights as the eldest.

REMEDIAL EDUCATION FOR THOSE WHOSE PERVERSE TENDENCIES ARE INSTINCTIVE

The instinctive, constitutional defect is most frequently associated with hereditary syphilis or alcoholism, and consanguinity of parents, malaria (which may have very serious consequences), broken or irregular homes. The mother has disappeared and been replaced by a step-mother, who shows herself indifferent, brutal or unjust. The father has left home, abandoning his wife and children (a frequent case) and the mother has rebuilt her life with another man who is jealous of the children of the first union and may himself be brutal and an alcoholic. The unfortunate children live in the streets, surrounded by bad examples, and wooed by depraved creatures of both sexes.

In all such tragic cases the remedial worker will have to draw not only on his great sense of mission, his skill and his highly-developed observation, but also on his profound and active sense of pity. Perversity is a precocious phenomenon. Hence the vital importance of applying remedial treatment as early as possible, as soon as the trouble is recognized. From his earliest years the perverse subject experiences the urge to do harm; his affective centre ceases to function; neither his parents nor the members of his family find favour in his sight. He is not amenable to any gesture of tenderness, goodness or forgiveness. The fear of a blow is equally without effect, since the child is skilful and knows how to protect himself.

In this perversity syndrome, the lie is king in a mythical world of false persuasion, accusation and calumny. The perverse subject steals, within the family circle, sweets, sugar, toys and finally money. Hypocrite, impostor and sneak, he is cruel, pinches, clutches, hides objects of everyday use, plays practical jokes, teases, tortures animals, and is neither obliging nor shows forethought. Fanatically self-centred, he has no time except for himself. In addition to this he breaks and destroys with immense pleasure. Sexual perversion forms part of this syndrome.

REMEDIAL EDUCATION
FOR THE PERVERSE* CHILD

1. On examination of the perverse child it is possible to establish his degree of opposition to authority which is the most usual sign of this defect. The first step is then to overcome this refusal to obey. This is the critical stage, on the result of which will depend the effect of future remedial treatment. Often the subject's opposition is manifested by a complete refusal to speak.

When the perverse child is being brought up in a good family environment by a mother ready to make every sacrifice to improve his condition, all is well and the teacher has a valuable assistant and partner. Where this is not the case after interviews with the parents and with the social worker, it is as well to consider placing the child in a school or foster home, where the climate will be more favourable for the development of his personality.

2. The first exercises to be performed are designed to achieve immediate obedience to precise orders. Orders should be given in a loud voice and no questions allowed. It is by means of the voice that the teacher makes his personality felt and obtains the compliance of the pupil.

3. Make the child carry out various very energetic co-ordination exercises, (upright position and horizontal on the back and on the stomach), in order to tire him out and by this means avoid sexual rages. Such sexual rages are in effect very common from the age of two years onwards and the only means of reducing their intensity is to produce a state of marked physical fatigue (the exercises should last half an hour morning and evening).

* This term no doubt includes those children usually described as maladjusted.

4. If the perverse child displays symptoms of aphasia (audio-mutism), exercises to alleviate mutism in aphasic children should be applied.

5. Arrange on the table a number of objects likely to arouse the covetous instincts of the child; toy car, lollipop, lump of sugar, coloured chalk, bar of chocolate, fruit, money, a small comb (it is advisable to find out in advance whether the child's preference is for objects (e.g. toys) or sweets), one or two pencils, etc.

6. Make the child recognize and call out the names of the objects (if the teacher has been able to provoke speech or if speech has returned owing to a weakening of opposition to authority).

7. Order the child to pick up one of the objects:

EXAMPLE:
Take a bar of chocolate.
Remove the paper.
Put it on the sideboard.

The child should be made to say each time, in succession:
(a) Oh what a lovely bar of chocolate!
(b) I am going to remove the paper.
(c) I am putting it on the sideboard.

8. The teacher gives the following orders:
Take the two shilling piece.
Put it in your pocket.
Give it to mother (or some third person).

Saying (in each case):
I am taking the two shilling piece.
I am putting it in my pocket.
I am giving it to mother.

9. At this stage the child should be made to do the following exercises (in the order shown) in the upright position with the arms stretched flat against the body:

1. Bend the knees.
2. Rise up straight again.
3. Turn the head (without moving the body) to the right.

4. Turn the head (without moving the body) to the left.

5. Return to the normal position.

6. Strike the thighs strongly.

10. Articulate in time with the above:
(If the child cannot talk, the vowels *ah–ee*, repeated alternately twelve times [the six movements to be carried out twice]); if the child can talk, repeat the words given below, in exact rhythm with the movements:

chocolate, sideboard, paper, two shillings, bar, pocket (words to be spoken from the first to the sixth then back to the first).

11. Order the child to replace the objects on the table in the order in which he originally took them, naming them one by one. The objects should be changed for each session.

12. If the child is very young—say three or four years old—the teacher may make him feel the effect of being pinched, scratched, bitten or having his possessions taken away; the teacher gives him a gentle pinch or bites him very lightly and takes some object out of one of the child's pockets.

In return he will let himself be pinched, scratched or bitten by the young defective, who is also allowed to remove an object from the teacher's pocket. The subject is made to say, as he attacks his teacher in the appropriate manner: *It is very bad to scratch, I must not bite* and (taking the stolen object) *I will not steal again.*

13. In between periods the teacher entrusts a sixpence to the pupil, or a handkerchief marked with his initials or some other object. This is to be brought back at the beginning of the next period.

14.(a) Such perverse children must also of course be taught good manners, e.g. to say: *Good-morning mother, Good-morning father, Good-morning Mrs. Jones* and in the same way, *Good-evening, Good-bye.*

(b) Articulate in very good time, to a beat of 4 (30 times a day): *It's bad to lie. I'll never lie again at all.*

15. The pupil should learn expressions imitative of satisfaction, hypocrisy and shame. This exercise is for children of the 6–8 age

group. Mimicry is a second language. It transmits the ideas suggested by words, developing the feeling in a manner that the words are incapable of expressing.

(a) Make the young liar articulate simple expressions.

EXAMPLE: *I am going to give Mummy a bunch of flowers.* This phrase should be spoken with a great outburst of joy, clapping the hands in great jubilation.

(b) Pronounce the same phrase with feeling and expression appropriate to a lie. Adopt an amused or embarrassed expression (the teacher should himself adopt such an expression as a stimulus for mimicry).

(c) The same phrase, pronounced with a feeling of despair, rage or shame at being caught out in a flagrant lie. Go through the same exercise 10 times, pointing out of course the stupidity, falseness and disgust inspired by a lie.

If the perverse subject suffers from language disorders, their removal by means of remedial treatment may markedly reduce the symptoms of perversity. The effect is one of liberation. If the child is an aphasic subject, recovery of the power of self-expression equally produces a feeling of release, a psycho-neural motor relaxation. If it is possible, moreover, effectively to interest the child in what goes on around him, this will also diminish his inclination toward cruelty and kleptomania, which can only be a sort of emotional transfer, a complex to avenge himself on his environment.

Corporal punishment is to be avoided. The exercise of a saintly patience toward the unfortunate child will lead him to regard his teacher as a haven of refuge, to feel at ease in his presence and obey him of his own free will.

This work requires stamina, skill and devotion. The prize is however a valuable one, when one remembers that, in working on the feelings and inclinations of perverse children, one is protecting society from the scourge of juvenile delinquency.

PERSONALITY DEFECTS

The character is the sum of tendencies some of which are inherent, while others are acquired from the environment. These tendencies toward certain types of action, which are in a constant state of flux, are composed of an essential basis of hereditary dispositions and of a series of external contributions of unequal value, which are constantly being renewed. The external contributions may balance or even outweigh the initial hereditary assets of the individual and acquire a governing influence on the behaviour of the child. If they are healthy and sound, a good balance is achieved; if they are morbid or of a harmful nature, the balance is disturbed. The personality of the child is marked by an extreme plasticity; it reacts at once to adapt itself to the environment, it is intensely sensitive to any moral shock, to examples set for him, to any variations in the climate of home or school. This explains the wide range of variation in the picture presented by the evolution of the child's personality: its lack of stability, its sudden depressions and equally sudden recoveries.

This plastic quality involves certain dangers, but at the same time gives us an opportunity to refashion or adapt the child's character. The hereditary tendencies are written too deep for erasure; they can, however, be canalized, strengthened, weakened, or neutralized by means of education, by means of psychic therapy, by contact with the outside world or by medical treatment. Together with the temperament and the constitution, the character makes up the sum total of the child's personality. Considered from a psychological aspect, the character is the index of the response of the individual, the temperament is the index of the response of the psychological system and the constitution is the index of the response of the physiological system (Laignel-Lavastine).

The phrases "defects of character", "distorted personality" are used to describe a further stage of development: perversity has become a more pronounced perversion. "Anti-social", "anti-authoritarian", "rebel", sometimes "paranoiac", "schizoid" and "cyclothymic" personalities with inclination toward theft, flight and especially lying, are the terms used to describe this state. The most serious cases are psychopaths, requiring specialist medical treatment. There are also children who express complete indifference, children who are depressed and children who are extremely disturbed. Those who suffer from defects of personality present a multiplicity of complex and involved symptoms. They constitute problems which appear insoluble even to the remedial worker. Remedial education is none the less to be recommended and should be applied in combination with the medical therapy.

Up to the age of five or six, such subjects are still regarded as perverse children. The critical period is that immediately following from six to puberty when the disturbances which emerge, in connection with the physical development of the individual, are aggravated by the problems of growth and of hormonal function.

This is where the teacher, the therapist, has a decisive role to play. From birth to puberty these subjects are first of all perverse children and only subsequently do they become distorted personalities. If they are treated in time, they become sound subjects with the possibility of a normal future, but if not, these unfortunates are predestined delinquents.

I shall never cease to say:

Treat the perverse child in time and the danger of delinquency need never arise.

This is a duty to humanity and to society, the vital importance of which should be plain to every eye.

How is one to ensure that it is accepted as such by the medical world, the public authorities and all who are responsible for the affairs of youth? The parents too, who should be the first to see that the proper steps are taken for the care of their children! Unfortunately they only too often "do not wish" to look the facts in the face, but prefer to deceive themselves with hope, piling up future sorrows for themselves and their children.

The points which require our careful attention are the character and the defects of the character. The character often includes noble qualities: pride, energy, will (sometimes taken for stubbornness), self-respect, inflexible loyalty. Adults of firm, unrelenting character, who are capable of dynamic efforts and great perseverance in the pursuit of their chosen aim, are often regarded as possessing "bad characters".

The same thing applies to children. One subject may have personality traits, which are considered shocking in the environment from which he springs. Against another family background, he might be regarded as having an interesting personality, endowed with intelligence and great possibilities for the future.

How many adolescents must be at loggerheads with their grandparents, parents, sisters, brothers and yet are far from being distorted personalities. Do their differences of opinion arise, for example, as a result of their interest in art, beauty or history? If they are growing up in a materialistic environment, hostile to such inclinations, they might easily be regarded as embittered characters, rebels against authority. There is really no end to the number of situations in which children may fail to be understood by their families.

For this reason whenever children of six or seven, or older, are brought to me with defects of character, established by test or observation, I feel it essential to examine the case with the most attentive care and with complete impartiality. One must study the environment in which the child is growing up, the forbears from whom he is descended and the races to which they belonged. One must try to obtain precise information on the atmosphere in the home, whether harmonious or not. A dossier of information on these lines will cast valuable light on the immediate environment of the child with a personality defect. Situations and circumstances can so often exist, which offend, distress and even wound the very soul of the young child.

Psycho-analytic methods, which have had such a vogue since the time of Freud are not in my view appropriate to such cases. The defects from which these children are suffering have often not been recognized by their families, or have been neglected. A slight hearing defect may have led to accusations of carelessness or stubbornness when the child fails to respond to a question or an order; some disability, dysphonia or dysarthria, which has not been discovered, may have hindered or disturbed the child's performance at school or behaviour at home. All these disabilities, which are closely linked to speech and hearing, are practically unknown to the psycho-analyst.

Slight attacks of stammering, which cause no concern to the family ("it will be all right", "it will cure itself"), may exercise an inhibitive effect on the child and cause him to withdraw into himself. The child is then said to be unsociable because he keeps himself to himself and avoids conversation. He thinks, he reflects, but he cannot express himself and give answers to questions. He prefers to keep silence ... This is then held against him ... he feels it, and appears to sulk. It is therefore worth paying some attention to the phonetico-auditory and psycho-cerebro-motor influences which affect the temperament, the reactions and the character of the child.

In the case of defects of this type the teacher should have recourse to the phonetic and psycho-neural motor remedial exercises, which I have described. A very striking type of defective personality is the unstable subject. Instability and constant agitation are usually accompanied by inability to concentrate and defects of judgement, intelligence and imagination (lying and lack of discipline). Often the unstable subject is afflicted with a "tic" of dystonic, sub-choreic, hypertonic or hypotonic origin, and he may also be given to biting his nails.

Thorough practice in retaining an immobile posture is the first step, together with psycho-neural motor training. Persevere with these exercises, with the deliberate intention of tiring the child, the only effective means of combatting the frequent sexual rages which occur. The exercises recommended in the case of those suffering from lack of motor co-ordination are particularly suitable for recalcitrant "tics" and nail-biting.

In addition to the psycho-neural co-ordination exercises, of which numerous examples can be drawn from the chapter devoted to stuttering, stammering and arhythmic stammering, the teacher should apply exercises involving judgement, rhythmic imagination and memory, which must be carefully synchronized with the body movements.

EXAMPLE: give the pupil twelve words, for which he is required to supply an adjective: *anger, quarrel, work, class, duty, order, effort, parents, table, hand-writing, lesson, reflection.* The child must find adjectives which fit these nouns.

Examples of suitable adjectives (given in the same order as the nouns): *unjust, stupid, useful, busy, sacred, clear, resolute, kind, polished, legible, interesting, deep.*

The nouns should then be learnt by heart with their adjectives, and recited in the order from one to twelve, then in the reverse order.

If the pupil is capable of doing so, he should be asked at each remedial session, to sit down at table and improvise a short conversation (on a different subject each time).

EXAMPLE 1: Your mother has asked you to do some shopping for her.

She has given you a list of what she wants (the pupil should be asked to make up a list of eight to ten different items).

Can you learn off the list by heart, repeat it back carefully and memorize it so as not to forget anything?

What would you choose if your mother told you to bring back some fruit, flowers or vegetables?

Make the child go through the names of fruit, flowers and vegetables which are in season.

Which shop would you go to for the various items?

EXAMPLE 2: What would you do if one of your friends fell down while playing and appeared to have hurt himself badly?

What would you do if your friend fell into a pond or a stream while out walking?

What would you do if he lost something?

How would you behave in these cases?

Your mother appears to be in pain or tired. How should you behave towards her? Would you be tempted to take advantage of her condition to be disobedient or would you help her by being as pleasant and helpful as possible?

EXAMPLE 3: You see that your brother, sister or friend has done something wrong. What would you do?

As can be seen, the teacher must constantly draw on his powers of imagination and adaptation in order to combine work on psycho-neural co-ordination with the psychic and mental training of the pupil and with the fostering of the mental and affective condition of the pupil.

Very frequently children with defects of the type described here are also nocturnal enuretics (bed-wetters). Up to the age of fifteen months the act of urination is an automatic reflex act, controlled only by the medulla. Between the ages of fifteen and twenty months, the normal child becomes clean as a result of the development of cortical control, thus gradually inhibiting the more elementary control exercised by the medulla. *Micturition becomes a controlled function.* If at three years the child continues to wet his bed, this is due to a functional retardation of the development of cortical control, the cause of which must be investigated. He has not acquired "urinary consciousness". This may be due to some local irritation (phimosis, malformation or stricture of the urinary duct, irritation of the genital or anal region). In such cases, or where the underlying causes are cortical or sub-cortical, medical care and treatment must be prescribed.

Various measures, which have proved effective, can however always be tried:

1. No liquid, soup, drink or fruit should be given to the child after 4 o'clock in the afternoon.

2. Since micturition tends to take place between 11 and 12 o'clock at night, the alarm clock should be set to go off at about 11 o'clock. The child wakes up, gets up, takes the chamber pot, empties its bladder, gets into bed and falls asleep again. If the child is able to carry out these movements on his own, no attempt should be made to watch him or speak to him.

3. If these measures prove effective, the alarm can be set progressively later. In this way we gain first an hour, then two hours, then more, and in the end the whole night. In this way the child or the adolescent acquires "urinary consciousness and discipline".

Children, grouped under the class heading "personality defects", suffer from a complex of deficiencies for which multisensory treatment must be given. The orthophonic specialist, when dealing with such cases, must make use of all his tact, skill, diplomacy, knowledge, observation, not to mention patience, intuition, intelligence and devotion. The placing of such young subjects in an institution is sometimes a good thing, provided the institution is well run and properly supervised; and always provided the numbers are not too great. If there is no family then the placing of the child in an institution is the only answer. The ideal solution, however, is and always will be for the child to remain within his family circle. Provided of course, that the mother accepts once and for all the advice of the remedial worker. An appeal must be made to the fullness of a mother's love.

Will not any mother, worthy of the name, always be ready to show heroic qualities of will-power, when it comes to a question of saving her child?

ANOREXIA

I have quite often come across children who systematically refuse all food. They display a profound aversion for all forms of nourishment, including cakes, chocolates and sweets, of which children are normally extremely fond.

Apart from the question of anorexia, such children seem normal, often even highly gifted intellectually. They speak and understand well and suffer from no serious defects of character. They are often smiling and friendly. The only indication of a psychopathological condition is their aversion to food.

I recently had under my care a delightful little girl of six, destined to be a dancer. Her movements came to her quite naturally and her dancing was already artistic; she had the gift of adapting her movements to the rhythm of the music. Her mother brought her to me in despair, because she would only consume an absurdly small quantity of food during the twenty-four hours. The little girl took an hour and a half to eat a quarter of a cutlet and secretly spat out any sweetmeats given to her, whenever she found a convenient opportunity. Persuasion, remonstrances, promises, rewards, nothing had any effect on this stubborn young person. Apart from this one point, she was easy to deal with, affectionate and charming.

Faced with this difficult case, I attempted to acquire an influence over the child by the power of the voice. My patient appeared sensitive in this respect: the spoken word seemed to move her.

1. I used this method of approach to make the child carry out very full respiratory movements in the lying position, with controlled expiration.

The child lies on his back on the floor.

Deep Inspiration	*Very rapidly:* breathe in silently with the nostrils dilated, no sniffing sound; the abdomen and the whole of the thoracic cage is expanded in one sharp movement.
Deep Expiration	*Very slow* movement: breathe out through the mouth; *very gently* drawing in the abdomen and the thoracic cage to the sound of the vowel *a*, while the teacher counts *slowly* from 1 to 20, then 1–25, 1–30 etc. Increase the duration each day.

This exercise is to be repeated twenty times per day. It should not be practised on a bed, but on the floor or on some other hard surface. The teacher counts the numbers out aloud, articulating clearly.

2. Lying flat on the floor, the child raises both arms and legs simultaneously, separates them, brings them together, saying very loudly, "I simply love hot buns" (One syllable per movement).

3. The same exercise is practised with the child saying twenty times, "The mayonnaise is simply lovely". As can be seen, it is perfectly possible to find phrases, like those above, which will

stimulate the appetite. The movements should also be varied and made as energetic as possible, in order to induce physical tiredness in the subject.

4. The teacher should have handy a roll, bun or some form of cake.

The child is instructed to go through the motions of chewing energetically but with the mouth empty (this should be timed half a second to the beat). The teacher controls the movement of the jaw, articulating at the same time clearly and loudly, "You are going to eat this cake" (at least 15 times) pointing to the cake in question.

5. Finally the teacher makes the pupil eat the cake, saying, "Chew it well! What you are eating is very good."

This phrase should be repeated over and over again, until the last morsel has gone down.

This technique is almost sure to be successful. Such is the effect of obedience to orders that I have even observed cases like the following: a patient suffering from anorexia got to the stage of asking for a bun or roll and starting to bite into it with gusto, even before coming into the presence of the remedial teacher. From then on all goes well and the anorexia subject regains weight and recovers mental calmness.

There exist forms of medical treatment for anorexia. Psychiatric research has led to discoveries in this field. My only aim here is to provide those working to help the defective child with details of a technique of remedial therapy which has in many cases given positive results.

CHILDREN WITH MULTIPLE DEFECTS WHO ARE EDUCABLE

Initial interview with the remedial teacher and sessions of appropriate remedial treatment

There are large numbers of defective children, who are neither victims of total aphasia, nor of motor defects, nor do they exhibit symptoms of serious mental deficiency. They are brought to us as a result of some single symptom, which is the despair of their parents, but is often the least serious symptom of a general syndrome. A persistent dysphonia or dyslalia may cause the family anxiety, without their paying particular attention to the marked psycho-motor instability. The child is not stupid, but finds it difficult to concentrate his mind, even for a few seconds, on a game or on something he has been told to do. Such children vary greatly in their initial reactions to the remedial teacher. As a teacher one must strive to avoid giving undue weight to the "first impression"; the dangers of being led astray in regard to treatment are too great.

The child often arrives laughing merrily and answers questions without hesitation. He seems to be trying to make an impression on his questioner. Everything comes easily to him, although his attention wanders to and fro like an imprisoned butterfly. If, however, the teacher follows his own plan of action and forces the young subject back into his final refuge, the little boy (or girl) will shy and "refuse" like a horse in front of a jump, and we get stamping of the feet, tears and opposition. This is the natural course of events, but it does not end there. If the teacher perseveres patiently, the child will begin to sense the presence of an inflexible authority and gradually becomes calmer and in a state of damp, tearful reserve performs the preliminary movements required for the remedial treatment. This is the inaugural session, which includes a careful examination of the child. In general we are faced with children who have become impossibly spoiled at home, since the parents, in fear of their paroxysms of rage, are afraid to cross their defective child.

Several periods are necessary in order to determine what should be the governing principles of the remedial treatment and where a start should be made. Several weeks will inevitably elapse before the child's possibilities, and his points of particular stubbornness can be assessed.

The parents also require to be trained. That is why I so strongly deplore the great weight now given to "tests". The indices on which the tests are based are related to the ages and physico-psychic characteristics of the child; they can thus constitute a source of error. These test results are assessments, which have been arrived at mathematically, and have nothing in common with the complex, unstable and, one might say, pathological natures of these defective children. Let these mathematical tests be applied to normal subjects. This may be accepted. In certain cases it may furnish valuable information. Even so one must be on the watch for the hypersensitive or inhibited individual.

The form of official snobbery which has for several years now insisted on the training of personnel qualified to apply these tests to children, would have been better employed in calling for the training of remedial teachers, capable of caring for defective children, freeing them from their fetters, helping them to join the column of humanity on the march, and, by means of unrelenting and devoted efforts, recreating in them human beings, capable of being of service to the family, to society, to the nation. This task, however, is difficult, wide in the scope of its application and quite exhausting. But what a fine ideal to pursue!

Sometimes the defective child tends to be timorous, fearful and ready to panic during the first interview. The presence of a remedial worker of either sex makes him think of a doctor or nurse and he recalls the needle. He must be cajoled, calmed and his confidence won. On other occasions we find ourselves faced by a subject who has deliberately retired behind a rampart of mutism. Our efforts to establish contact remain fruitless. The child studiously avoids the eye of this passing interrogator. This state of complete quiescence requires a modification of tactics, but success can always be achieved in the end. In cases of this sort, where tangible opposition can be felt, it is a good thing to get the subject away from the parents or those who represent parental authority. This move may produce different reactions in the child: he may cry with all his might or fly into a sudden rage, or he may immure himself even deeper in his stubbornness. At this point, for all the cases which I have just described, the controlled movements of the co-ordination exercises can have a decisive effect.

1. Gently, but with unshakeable firmness, lay the child on his back on the floor. In spite of tears, rages or other forms of oppo-

sition, make the child carry out the controlled movements of raising and lowering the legs, then the arms, counting loudly, One! Two! Three! Four! The teacher kneels on the ground, of course, beside the angry child.

2. Next vary the movements: open the legs, cross them, open again, then the same movements with the arms, articulating at the same time the names of various articles, which can be opened and crossed like the legs and arms: scissors, pincers, penknives, points. If the child is incapable of understanding the allusion, use the names of toys and familiar objects (soap, sponge, towel, tap).

The important thing is for the teacher to raise her voice. This is an extremely important element in the process of calming the panic-striken subject. The voice can exercise a very considerable influence on the psychic state of the child: it can impress, calm, win over the little one. After the conclusion of this infallible method of calming the child, the parents may be brought back into the room.

The child is now at ease, smiling and watching the teacher with a sort of amused distrust. The phonetic examination may now be undertaken.

3. When assessing the auditory receptivity and ability to articulate, the teacher should try to make the child imitate the phonetic sounds of consonants, carefully noting any altered or deficient sounds. Begin with the consonants associated with the vowel *a*, which should be treated in the following way: make the child repeat: *ba ka da fa* (*ka* sometimes tends to become confused with *da* and the *f* may be deficient).

ga ja cha la ma na pa ra sa ta va xa (ksa) ya za

The consonants most likely to be affected are: the fricatives, — including *sh* and *zh* (as in *pleasure*) — the gutturals, the sibilants, sometimes the lingual *l* and the dentals.

4. Check whether or not any of the following dysphonias exist: open or closed rhinolalia or hoarseness (always possible).

5. Make the child pronounce simple words; note any inversions, or sounds that are suppressed or confused.

6. Any choreic movements or symptoms of adiadochokinesis should be noted.

7. Ask the child to place his hands on the table and to separate the fingers and bring them together again. Can he do this?

8. If the child is in a state of constant movement, get him to stand upright with the arms and legs apart, with his eyes trained on the teacher. He should be kept in this position while the teacher counts slowly in a loud voice from 1 to 20 or 30 and then from 20 or 30 to 1. This is very important, since the defective child finds this unusual method of counting upwards and downwards astonishing, even if he does not fully understand it, and remains riveted in his position.

9. Where the child's intelligence is sufficiently alert, he may be asked to give the names of four-legged and two-legged animals and the names of the seasons, the months and the days of the week.

10. The teacher should now test the child's knowledge of his own person, asking him to indicate his right and left arms, waist, chest, etc.

This is a plan for the observation of the child at the initial interview, but it is capable of considerable variation. One must in fact proceed as best one can, suiting the method to the motor, cerebral and phonetic characteristics of the child and to the traits of his personality. Also to be taken into account is the mentality of the mother or the person responsible for the child. The plan can be used as a guide, but must subsequently be adapted to the particular circumstances.

REMEDIAL SESSIONS FOR THE CHILD WITH TOTAL OR PARTIAL DEFECTS

Notes must be made at each session, whether weekly, bi-weekly or tri-weekly, of the exercises to be practised at home; this may be done in an ordinary school note-book, which should be brought by the mother no later than the second session.

1. Exercises designed to reduce the subject's opposition to authority and make him obey simple orders. Example: moving

articles from one position to another, picking up a watch, putting it on the table, giving it to his mother, putting it back in its normal place.

Take a book, open it, shut it, move it around, put it back in its original place. Sometimes the mother interrupts the lesson in the following way: "You can see, Mrs.—— that he (or she) can do it all. *He understands everything*" (the last phrase is repeated over and over again). "As soon as his father comes home, he goes and fetches his slippers, etc."

The teacher must not be put off by this, but must carry on with the exercises, pointing out that the actions which the child carries out instinctively or of his own free will, do not possess the same value as actions performed in obedience to the will of the teacher, since the latter indicate a slackening of the child's opposition to authority.

2. Where the child is continually in movement, tiring himself and his family with this incessant, pointless activity, the teacher should persevere with the immobility exercises. These are key exercises both for their calming effect and for fostering stability in the subject.

Put the child in the following position: upright, legs together, arms outstretched "to the rear" with the hands well stretched and the body leaning forward so as to bring the head down to the level of the knees.

The teacher should insist on complete physical immobility counting up to 30, 40 and 50 and then back from 50 to 1 (this exercise to be carried out 6 times).

3. Reverse position: upright, leaning backwards and looking up at the ceiling. Arms and hands should be stretched forwards with the hands outstretched, not clenched. Same period of immobility (6 times).

4. Upright, arms outstretched horizontally, feet together; raise one leg as high as possible and bend the knee; attempt to remain stationary in this position, which is not an easy task, since static equilibrium of these children is weak. Initially they may be allowed to support themselves with the tip of the index finger on the back

of a chair. Practise the same exercise with each leg. The duration of this exercise should be initially adjusted to suit the motor capacity of the pupil. Subsequently the duration can be gradually increased.

5. The child is made to lie on the ground, supporting the weight of the upper part of the body on the fore-arms, in imitation of the "sunbathing" position.

Slowly lift the outstretched legs 12 to 18 inches off the ground. Remain immobile in this position (very difficult to achieve), while the teacher counts. The exercise should be continued up to the pupil's limit of endurance (repeat 5 times).

6. Reverse position: half-lying, half-sitting, legs extended on the ground, arms and hands stretched out in front. Count during the exercise and each day increase its duration. (Repeat the exercise five times in succession).

Using these fundamental exercises as a starting point, it is easy to invent others, suited to the physical and cerebral characteristics of the pupil.

7. When the child's opposition (by the end of two or three sessions) has to some extent worn down, the immobility exercises can be practised with spoken comments by the pupil (these are highly beneficial even for normal subjects suffering from excessive nervousness). They should, for example, be made to adopt a position such as this: upright, one arm raised slightly above the horizontal, one slightly lowered. The child is then instructed to repeat 20 times in a loud voice with clear articulation phrases like the following: "I must sit still in class" or "I must not move at all" or "I must look people in the face, when they are talking to me".

The voice should be rather loud with rhythmic articulation, syllable by syllable, with an appropriate timing of a quarter second per syllable.

8. If the educable defective child is an aphasic patient, or if he is subject to phonetic or language disorders, reference should be made to the chapter which is devoted to remedial phonetic education.

9. The following exercises should be performed in those very frequent cases where the child pronounces "krain" instead of "train" and "totolate" instead of "chocolate" or "tow" instead of "cow".

Work at the syllables: *tera, teray*, etc. then *tera, kra, dera, gra*, etc.

10. In the sitting position, provided the child is sufficiently advanced mentally, practise the following exercise: strike the table with both hands, saying "palm", then turn them over saying "back".

When this has been done, practise striking the hands on the table, one with palm, the other with the back, strictly in time together, shouting: right palm, left back, left palm, right back (at least 20 times in succession).

11. In those cases where at the first examination the child is noticed to suffer spasmodic movements or "tics", it is most important to proceed in the way described below.

The "tic" is the continued repetition of a gesture or attitude, which is *prima facie* perfectly normal. The abnormal element is the repetition of this gesture or attitude without valid justification at the behest of some compulsion that will not be denied.

After observing carefully the nature and context of this spasmodic movement, it should be broken down into two or three separate movements according to the individual case and practised slowly.

EXAMPLE: A child blinks incessantly.

Make the child close his eyes, so that the eyelashes disappear, then open them, raising the eyebrows fully (this exercise to be practised to a beat of two, clapped with the hands). Strict time must be observed.

The child suffers from a spasmodic movement of the neck or shoulders, or of one shoulder. The "tic" should be broken down into two or three components and these movements carried out in the appropriate time. I knew of one case where the child, as soon as a new phrase had been learnt, rubbed the inside of one knee against the other and then separated the legs sharply. He was cured in six weeks by practising this movement in six time. Three beats on the knees, three beats on the shoulders, counted out slowly. The disparity between the vertical movement of the hands and the horizontal movement of the legs contributed greatly to this cure.

CHAPTER V

CHILDREN WITH SENSORY DEFECTS

DEAFNESS, SEMI-DEAFNESS AND SLIGHT HEARING DEFECTS

I feel it is worth recalling something of the history of the alleviation of mutism in deaf people. It is of interest for remedial workers to know what has been done, and what has been left undone in the past on behalf of these people, deprived of one of their senses but in all other respects normal, often highly intelligent and worthy above all of care, of a scientifically based education and devoted attention.

Many centuries had to pass before the deaf won the right to receive instruction, to earn their living and enjoy the privileges accorded to every citizen. In Greece, in the city state of Sparta, before the time of Jesus Christ, they were still a long way from this: those with defective hearing were required to disappear. In certain parts of Gaul, they were sacrificed to pagan deities. In Rome the deaf were deprived of the rights of citizenship; they were obliged to accept a guardian to look after their affairs. How unfortunate were the deaf in ancient times! They were unkindly dealt with by the writers; Pliny regarded them as idiots; Lycurgus condemned them to death. Aristotle and Hippocrates despised them. Later in medieval times, the deaf were considered as madmen and as such were isolated. No one bothered about them. Only in the 16th century do we find any better understanding of the state of those with auditory defects. The first attempts at the education of deaf-mutes were made in Spain by a Benedictine monk, named Ponce de Léon (1520–1584) and by Ramirez de Carrion. In 1620 Pablo Bonet d'Aregon wrote a treatise on the teaching of speech. In 1700 a doctor, in practice in Holland, Conrad Hamman, made a determined assault on the problem of the education of deaf-mutes. He was followed by Ernaud and Pereire (1760) and the Abbé Deschamps; in Scotland by Thomas Braidwood; in Germany by Heinike. The latter founded at Leipzig in 1778 a school where speech training had priority amongst the teaching methods (natural gestures, manual alphabet, lip-reading). This method, called the German method, was in fact nothing more than the reappearance of the method which had for a long time been used in Spain, in Scotland, in Holland and especially in France.

In France during the period which overlapped the end of the eighteenth and the beginning of the nineteenth century, three names stand out: two priests, the Abbé de l'Épée and the Abbé Sicard and a doctor, Dr. Itard.

The Abbé de l'Épée (1712–1789) had opened a school in his own house. There he held sessions three times a week for deaf mutes, living with their families, and for others, who were housed at his expense in neighbouring lodgings. To this generous cause he devoted his fortune, his intelligence and his vocation as priest. He was able to bring his influence to bear on the élite of Parisian society to such an extent that even members of the Royal Family came to watch his work.

As is generally known the Abbé de l'Épée was the inventor of the system of sign language which remained in use among teachers of deaf-mutes up to 1880. This did not mean that he was opposed to the principle of speech training by means of the spoken word, the fundamental principle of the oral method. He well understood the importance of the spoken word as a complementary form of instruction for deaf mutes. Was it not in fact de l'Épée who wrote that "the only method of bringing back the deaf mute into society is to teach him to hear with his eyes and speak with his human voice? The world will never learn to talk with fingers and eyes for the pleasure of conversation with deaf mutes".

Initially when his pupils were few, he attempted to make them speak, but he was gradually overwhelmed by the ever-increasing numbers of his pupils and he eventually renounced this method of instruction in favour of sign language. However this may be, his work remains of eternal value, since with him opens the era of redemption for deaf mutes. After his death the National Constituent Assembly placed him among the ranks of "those citizens who have deserved best of their country and of humanity". His reputation survived the tormented time of the Revolution.

Successor to the Abbé de l'Épée was another priest, the Abbé Sicard, the second centenary of whose birth was celebrated in 1942 by all deaf mutes in France. The Abbé Sicard was born at Fousseret in the Department of Haute-Garonne on September 20th 1742. He studied and was ordained at Toulouse. Arriving in Paris in 1785 he studied the Abbé de l'Épée's method for the education of deaf mutes, under de l'Épée himself. He then became director of the school for deaf mutes which had just been founded at Bordeaux, and remained there until the death of the Abbé de l'Épée. He was then summoned to Paris to succeed this great benefactor of deaf mutes.

The National Constituent Assembly raised the schools in Paris and Bordeaux to the rank of National Institutions. The Paris school was established in the old Saint-Magloire Seminary in the Faubourg St. Jacques, where it still exists.

"I have discovered the glass" said the Abbé de l'Épée to Sicard, "you must make the spectacles". Several years later the Abbé Sicard spoke of the Abbé de l'Épée in the following words: "As for myself, who have the honour to be his immediate successor, who have been a witness to his zeal and whom he charged, on his deathbed, to continue his work, if I have been able to add to his noble foundations, if I have extended and perfected his sublime discovery, I must state that I have only worked for the glory of a master, so justly famed, and to whom must be ascribed any credit there is in what I have been able to do."

In spite of the revolution and its attendant dangers Sicard devoted himself to his task with faith and enthusiasm. He seemed to put more trust in the art of mime than in spoken language. There is little doubt, however, that he must have regarded the system of sign language, practised and recommended by him, as a necessity, rather than a final, exclusive answer, since the Abbé Sicard, like the Abbé de l'Épée, lacked the trained personnel necessary to carry out oral instruction.

The Abbé Sicard had a prodigious capacity for work; he was a walking encyclopaedia. He was, moreover, a teacher at the École Normale Supérieure and a member of the Académie Française. He was a great priest, a great thinker, a great apostle.

The Abbé Sicard had the good fortune to encounter the man who was destined, as a result of prolonged experimentation, remarkable perseverance in the cause of science and a profound study of the nature of the deaf mute and of otology in general, to pave the way for the introduction in the distant future of the oral and acoustic method of education for deaf mutes. His name was Itard.

Itard, a French doctor, was born at Oraison (Basses-Alpes) in 1775 and became a pupil of Larrey and Pinel. He turned aside from general surgery in order to carry his investigations into the little-known field of diseases of the ear. It was Itard who pioneered the opening of the tympanum in the case of infection of the middle ear and the catheterization of the Eustachian tube. He entered the field of the education of deaf mutes under the direction of the Abbé Sicard and set himself to work on the problem of aural instruction. The name of this doctor is indissolubly linked with the oral method of acoustic education, of which he was the real creator.

In spite of the official support of the Academy of Medicine (6 May 1828), in spite of the initiative of Itard and the untiring efforts of the director and all the teaching personnel, the oral method of instruction did not obtain an acknowledged position in this establishment until October 18th 1880. Up to that date it was only dealt with in a supplementary course.

In about 1910 at Rouen, Dr. Tillot made use of an acoustic tube of his own design in attempts to awaken auditory perception in various deaf mute cases and to improve the hearing of patients with acquired deafness. In 1924 a further step forward was taken, this time in the field of specialized instruction. Dr. Decroly devised in Belgium his so-called global method of education, which was taken up by Professor Herlin of the Institute for Deaf Mutes in Paris. I cannot forbear to mention that Gérard de Parrel devoted to the cause of the deaf, during the first half of this century, the best of his studies and of his medical activities. In his especial devotion to the cause of deaf children he was for them the great successor and apostle of de l'Épée and Sicard, of Itard and Tillot.

At the present time optimum conditions exist for the social rehabilitation of deaf mutes provided they receive remedial education in their family right from the "earliest age". It is possible for their residual auditory capacity to be trained and developed by appropriate exercises and for them to be trained in a manual craft or a profession suited to their capabilities.

Some deaf people, who have received remedial education have been able to reach high positions: for example, a patient with a severe degree of congenital deafness was accepted at the École des Chartes, where he did extremely well and at present occupies an important executive position.

It is wrong to think that severely deaf people are only capable of unimportant and manual activities. Where the subjects are intelligent and talented, they are able to make their way in the liberal professions: engineers, chemists, scientists of all types, all of course in professions where their deafness does not constitute a special handicap. They get married, produce children and very often the children hear perfectly.

We are concerned here with the deaf only in regard to remedial education of the baby. Only the doctor is qualified to diagnose the numerous underlying causes of deafness and prescribe the appropriate treatment.

The audiogram can provide precise information on the degree of bilateral hearing deficiency. Aural surgery can today claim positive results, nor do I need to describe the tremendous help that some deaf subjects have received from hearing aids.

In spite of the progress of science, however, whose frontiers are steadily being extended throughout the world, the deaf person is still largely dependent on remedial education. Nothing will ever be able to provide a complete substitute for individual remedial treatment carried out in accordance with modern methods and applied constantly and methodically.

Once medical authority has been obtained, along what lines should the remedial teacher attempt to proceed?

1. *From the age of eight to ten months* he should attempt to stimulate and develop the residual auditory capacity.

2. He should make methodical use of lip-reading in order to produce speech, ensuring at the same time that the deaf child should develop an audible voice and clear articulation, and acquire a knowledge of words.

3. He should prepare the child early to attend school; the deaf child needs to have a start on hearing children and should, if possible, from the age of four onwards, be familiar with the terms in most common use at school. At least a half of those children who are deaf possess residual auditory capacity to a more or less significant degree. Advantage must be taken of this. Some of them are able to perceive the sound of the voice when contact is made with their outer ear and some distinguish a variation in vocal timbre. Others show very little reaction to the sound of the voice. Some can only be reached by sounds of high intensity, such as those emitted by an alarm clock, whistle or by instruments designed to produce sounds varying in intensity and pitch. Some can only perceive sounds of certain pitches within the tonal scale; they have auditory islands.

With very young children there can be no question of audiometric procedures. We can only use the human voice, whistles, clocks or tuning forks to produce palpebral or otocephalogyric responses. No account should be taken of reflexes provoked by the transmission of sound through solid media, vibrations along the floors or walls, resulting from the slamming of a door or a blow struck against a table or wall. This may be mistaken for auditory perception but it is essentially tactile in origin. The aim is to teach the subject to differentiate vocal sounds, using voice and microphone amplifiers. Very useful instruments of this type have been designed during the past few years.

Good results can be achieved with young deaf children by the use of extremely loud, voiced sounds. This should be done as soon as the deficiency is noted, i.e. as soon as possible before the end of the "first year".

The deaf child has everything to gain by remaining with his family, taking part in the events of everyday life, struggling to understand and to make himself understood by means of the spoken word. Sign language should be disregarded. This is the ideal but we must, of course, take account of the hazards and difficulties of life with the family; fortunately there do exist a number of schools and institutions which take a limited number of pupils, where the children can receive individual treatment and tuition. Such institutions are, however, few. There remain finally the Institutions for deaf mutes, which must cater for excessive numbers of pupils. The specialized attention which deaf patients require is admittedly provided, but everything becomes difficult when the number of pupils is too great for the teaching personnel. In any case no institution can accept a child which is only a few months old. At this age only the mother and the family can undertake the care of the deaf baby. It is moreover at this age that the deaf child must be prepared for hearing. Such children, who seem at first quite beyond the reach of sounds, are sometimes able, after months of patient acoustic exercises, to perceive rudimentary auditory impressions. It is of vital importance to help the child with impaired hearing. He will reap the benefit all his life, so that the result justifies any effort.

I give below a series of exercises designed to be given to the child from the age of a few months up to 18 months. That is to say at the vital age from the point of view of the preparation for the education of deaf children.

EXERCISES

Exercise 1: On the advice and with the authority of the medical specialist, carry out vocal vibrations close to each ear, using a rolled *r*. This exercise should produce "cascades of sound". Each sound should be attacked "mezza voce", rising through a "crescendo" to "forte" and then gradually diminishing. This exercise should be carried out 25 times for each ear, 4 times per day. Only the devotion of a mother's heart can achieve such a precise effort over a period that may extend to years. Patience and stamina are needed.

The reactions of the deaf child must be observed with the closest attention. In general the child appears to find this exercise pleasant. Sometimes he is frightened and starts to cry, but this does not last long and he rapidly gets used to the exercises.

The consonant *r* may be associated initially with the vowel *ee*. The vibrant syllables may then be practised in turn: *rrrrree rrrray rrrroo rrrroa (boat)*.

It is easy to establish, by watching the baby's reactions whether one vowel is heard better than another. Special stress is then placed on the vowel that can be heard.

Sometimes the vowel *ee* carries better to the child than *ah*. Intonation and sex exercise an influence on the position of vocal sounds in the tonal scale: female voices are more high-pitched than male. On the other hand the composition of a particular word may affect its audibility, according to whether high or low-pitched sounds predominate, therefore the different vocal levels need to be taken into account in acoustic measurement and in remedial education.

Is it necessary to point out that these acoustic exercises must be carried out with maximum resonance in the voice? There are voices which are devoid of all timbre, power and vibrato. For the deaf child this is disastrous. It should be possible, though, to call on someone in the child's circle with the right type of voice. It is possible to use musical or other sound-producing instruments as a substitute, but in fact nothing is as good as the vibrations of the human voice to reanimate the acoustic nerve of the deaf child.

Exercise 2: Increase the range of the "cascades of sound" by the vibrant pronunciation of other syllables, including the vibrant *r*, so as to accustom the deaf child to make use of its ears and differentiate the vocal sounds. If the child is allowed to remain in the grip of his auditory deficiency, he will never suspect that the function of hearing exists. It must be demonstrated to him that the ear is an organ which he can use.

The following vowels should be pronounced with great vocal power close to each ear, prolonging the sound: *e* (repeated) as in *bet*, then *ay*, then *ee, er, oo, wa.*

Each vowel sound should be drawn out for approximately a second, the whole exercise repeated 6 times. Sometimes, at the end of a varying period of time, the baby manages to reproduce instinctively the sound he hears. One should not mistake the value of this small victory. It is not a miracle. Miracles are, alas, not ours to command. We are only attempting to add a little bit to the acoustic capital of the deaf child and establish the precise discrimination of certain vocal sounds, in such a way that the child becomes conscious, as far as is possible, of the intonation and rhythm of the spoken word.

The psychic tendencies, character traits and nervous condition of the subject may on occasion make it difficult to carry out these exercises. The baby, if it is agitated, throws itself about, cries (because deaf children cry a lot). If it proves difficult to calm the baby, the love of the mother may be displayed on its side and with all the stubbornness of which she is capable. This situation requires the patience of a saint; the vital thing is that the treatment should go on. In nine cases out of ten, where the child is normal the automatic reactions of an acquired discipline will prove soothing. The exercise should be practised with complete precision. They should if possible be carried out at fixed times (3 times per day).

Exercise 3: Auditory orientation by means of exercises to practise the localization of the sources of sounds of varying resonance.

The child is placed in the middle of a room, where someone plays with him to distract his attention. The teacher rings a bell, sounds the alarm of a clock, a siren, a horn if she has one, or plays a musical instrument; chords, in the base or treble, on the piano or harmonica, trumpet or flute, may be sounded from different directions in the room or from the next room.

The person playing with the child watches his auditory reflexes to see whether there is even an approximate orientation toward the source of the sound.

This exercise to be repeated every day.

Exercise 4: The teacher should aim as far as possible at producing auditory adaptation to the following syllables (to be repeated in groups of 3 in each of the child's ears): *pa! ba! ma!* (six times), *lala leelee lon-lon, fa fo foo, gree gran grwa, vro vroo vrer, kru kron krin, jasha shojo jushu, seze seezee san zan, raya rooyoo royo, da ta na, di ti ni, du tu nu.*

Four of these groups of syllables should be called loudly every day in each ear of the deaf child.

I shall never cease proclaiming the truth that the deaf child (who is a normal child) has a right to be taught to speak. If the deaf child cannot speak at the same age as other children, then he will be a "frustrated" creature, since the deaf need not be mute. He does not speak simply because he cannot hear; it is up to those of his family circle to teach him to speak at the age normal for the acquisition of phonetic speech, i.e. toward eighteen months old. Families and children's nurses must be clear about this. A deaf child, possessing normal mental equipment, but unable to speak, is a neglected, abandoned, frustrated being, a heart-rending victim of the ignorance of those responsible for him. I am well aware that the teaching of deaf children can be infinitely laborious, but it is a duty, a duty owed in the name of humanity, of the family, of society. No one should be allowed to shirk it. Never should the deaf child be allowed to become in that repulsive but common expression, a "deaf mute". If he does, he has every right to harbour a grievance for all his coming years against those whose negligence ignorance and laziness have brought this to pass.

Efforts should be directed toward making the production of speech simultaneous with attempts at reanimating the acoustic nerve. At this initial stage lip-reading is a manifestation of voluntary attention and develops visual perception. One can see here how tremendously valuable it can be to familiarize the child, right from the beginning, with vocal sounds. If he has learnt to differentiate even approximately a few sounds, this is an inestimable advantage in regard to his more rapid initiation into the problems of articulation.

Close attention by the child to the movements of the teacher's mouth is the direct road to speech. We can add to this purely visual and external aid, the information afforded by the feel of the organs of speech: tongue, larynx (thryoid cartilage, nostrils, cheeks, lips, teeth).

It is common practice to speak of the deaf child exactly as if it could hear. Subjects with hearing defects gradually acquire a wonderful ability to decipher the designs made by the lips, the various words and phrases. For example, the child may learn to say "Daddy" and "Mummy" very young, having read these sounds on the lips. Parents sometimes take this for auditory assimilation of the sound. It is nothing of the sort.

Speech is not only a question of muscular movements; it is accompanied by respiratory and vibratory phenomena, which vision alone without touch, cannot fully grasp. For those unfortunate children, who are not only deaf, but blind, the sense of touch is the one key to education. There are some very wonderful women who have specialized in this particularly delicate and difficult form of remedial education. They sometimes achieve very surprising results. It is true of course that everything depends on the intellectual, psychic and cerebral receptivity of the child. Some respond rapidly to the stimulus of education, others more slowly, some again are stubborn, limited in their powers of understanding and negative in their attitude to the work. Even in these more serious cases, it is worthwhile to persevere, in the expectation of a cerebral awakening that may occur at any moment.

Exercise 5: The teacher should place himself squarely in front of the child and in a good light in such a way that no aspect of his articulatory movements escape the pupil.

(a) First he articulates very loudly, close to the ear of the child, the syllable *ba*, then he demonstrates the plosive element in this syllable against the child's hand (the child must be made to watch the whole procedure with close attention). The child is then asked to articulate the syllable energetically against his own hand. The child will often perform the articulatory movement without producing a sound. In such a case, the teacher repeats the process, drawing out the vowel, and then calls it in the ear of the deaf child who will eventually produce a voiced sound.

By 18 months or 2 years at the latest, when maximum reanimation of the acoustic nerve has been achieved, we get a clear voice without the monotonous guttural intonation which is so unpleasant to hear.

Once the auditory and phonetic adaptation are combined, the deaf child acquires, for the rest of its life, a voice that is audible and less distorted than that of his fellows in misfortune. All the more reason to ensure that the process of acoustic stimulation is begun before the baby reaches the age of one.

(b) As soon as the syllable *ba* has been mastered, both in regard to lip-reading and articulation, it should be practised with all the vowels in turn, the teacher demonstrating energetically the positions of the mouth to show the external differences between the various vowel sounds.

bay open the mouth wide, separating the corners of the lips.

bee the commissures of the lips are opened to the fullest extent. If necessary the cheek muscles should be forced back by hand to indicate the high-pitched sound.

bo! the child should be made to appreciate the difference between the *o* in *bottle* and the *o* in *boat*, by feeling with his finger the roundness of the lips during the explosion of this syllable.

bew (as in *beau*tiful) this is less easy to demonstrate. It must be attempted several times from the starting point *bee*, so as to indicate the difference in the position of the labial muscles. Above all try to bring home to the child the difference in auditory timbre.

boo the articulation of this syllable is relatively easy to achieve, pouting and folding the lips as if to whistle.

bwa this vowel must be practised in two separate parts, *boo...a,* slurred together. Refer to the indications given above regarding this vowel.

ber a more complicated sound to imitate. The consonant should explode with the lips well forward, the sound to be perceived by each ear.

bwee separate the sounds into *boo...ee,* advancing the lips for the *ee* sound, then returning them to the normal position.

All the above consonants and vowels must be mastered initially in the "strong" position, then in the "weak" position, then in the inter-vocalic position and finally within the framework of words. This principle must always be observed. I state it here once and for all.

Exercise 6: We are now left with the unvoiced consonant *pa,* which is achieved by labial explosion on to the hand of teacher and pupil, who must then be made to feel by placing his hand on the teacher's neck, the laryngeal vibrations, produced by *b,* but not by *p.* Tireless repetition of these two movements will produce perfect differentiation between the pronunciation of these two consonants. The consonant *p* should then be practised with all the vowels, given above, using lip-reading techniques.

Exercise 7: The development of the unvoiced and voiced gutturals (velar plosives) *ka* and *ga.*

(a) by means of the tactile sensation received by the pupil's hand placed first against the neck of the teacher, then against his own, the pupil is brought to perceive the sensation of throat clearance at the back of the throat (40 times per period).

(b) mouth wide open, tongue pressed against the base of the mouth by means of a tongue-depressor, develop the sound *ka;* repeat the exercise as often as necessary for the acquisition of the sound. Much attention must be given to this, the acquisition of this sound being very often a measure of the effort made by the teacher. Use of the tongue-depressor should be discontinued as soon as possible.

Exercise 8: Acquisition of the sound *ga* in exactly the same way as for the preceding exercise. The pupil's hand should be placed further down the neck, in order to feel the vibration of the larynx.

Exercise 9: Practise these two sounds and in order to make them appreciable to the lip-reader, place the pupil's hand low down the neck, so as to demonstrate the articulation. The teacher can obtain this immediate transfer by placing his hand lightly at the level of his own larynx. The two gutturals *k* and *g* should of course be practised both in regard to lip-reading and articulation*, in association with all the vowels listed at the beginning of this study.

Exercise 10: Development of articulation and recognition through lip-reading of the consonants *f* and *v*.

Using the hand, make the child bite his lower lip. Holding this position, he should then blow as hard as possible. In general these sounds are very easy to read on the lips of the teacher and to imitate. The child is able to differentiate between the two sounds as a result of the presence of laryngeal vibration with *v* and its absence with *f*. These consonants should then be practised through the vowel range, for lip-reading and articulation simultaneously. In addition of course, these sounds should be practised for lip-reading and articulation in the strong, weak and intervowel positions.

Exercise 11: Development of articulation and recognition through lip-reading of the voiced and unvoiced fricatives *zh* (as in plea*s*ure) *sh*. The child finds it fairly easy to master these sounds. He lip-reads them and is able to appreciate by touch the changes taking place in the phono-articulatory organs (lips, tongue, larynx, dental arches and cheeks), the vibratory movements that may echo along them, the production of heat, the shape and force of air emission and the function of the nasal and buccal orifices in the emission and articulation of certain vocal sounds.

* It must be realized that very little of the movements which produce *k* and *g* are visible to the lip-reader.

Apart from the active tactile sensation, resulting from the presence of the pupil's fingers on the speech organs of the teacher or on his own, there is also a sort of "inner sense of touch", whereby the child is able to feel the vibrations that are produced in these organs. In the case of a gifted child, this creates a sort of automatic function of the memory and motor apparatus, which develops with the acquisition of different sounds.

As regards these fricative consonants, the teacher clenches his teeth, protrudes his lips and blows on the child's hand:

shsh   shsh   shsh

The child is quick to imitate this movement as it is plainly visible.

He clenches his teeth.
He protrudes his lips.
He blows strongly behind his teeth.

Difficult as this exercise is to achieve correctly in the case of psychic or mental deficiency, it can very easily be mastered by a deaf child of normal intelligence.

To amuse the child, little piles of paper can be blown across the table during the exercise. As in previous cases these consonants should not be articulated initially with vowels. Articulation and lip-reading can be mastered more quickly if the vowels and consonants are kept separate

shsh .... *a*
shsh .... *ay* etc.

Once the vowels separated in this way from the consonants have been achieved continue with *sha, shay, sho* (as in *pot*), *shoo, shwa, shwee.* I must stress again that lip-reading and articulation must be practised with the consonants in both the strong and weak positions: *in front of the vowel, after the vowel* and *within the word.*

EXAMPLES: *ash, aysh, eesh, osh,* etc.

The same technique is applied for the voiced consonant, making the child feel the laryngeal vibrations.

Exercise 12: The lingual *l* is also quick to be learnt and pronounced by the normal deaf child.

1. The following procedure is sufficient:

(a) Open the mouth.
(b) Put out the tongue without closing the mouth.
(c) Close the mouth.

2. The teacher, starting with the explosive *ba*, pushes out the tip of the tongue and lets it vibrate against the outer face of the lips.

ba   llllll

The infant generally finds this an amusing game and is happy ₜo imitate it (60 times per day).

3. If articulation of this sound is slow in coming, make use of a tongue-depressor. It is placed vertically in the front of the mouth of the infant who puts out his tongue to reach it. This very simple procedure is decisive in nine cases out of ten. Combination of the *l* with the vowel sounds and lip-reading normally present no difficulty.

Exercise 13: The sibilants *s* and *z* are sometimes rather long in coming. The teacher demonstrates as follows:

(a) Clench the teeth.
(b) Open the lips.
(c) Whistle *se* behind the teeth, dealing with the unvoiced consonant first.
(d) The child's finger is placed on the incisors of the teacher, so as to bring home to him the sibilant effect.

This exercise should be practised as often as is required to achieve correct articulation of this sound. Lip-reading should also be practised, of course, and the consonant should be made as audible as possible, in conjunction with the range of vowels.

The voiced consonant presents less difficulty since it is more obvious and if it has been possible to develop any residual auditory capacity, it can be heard.

These consonants, by contrast with the others, may be combined with vowels right away. They form a common entity. They may, therefore, be articulated and recognized by means of lip-reading directly:

sa say see so soo swa ser swee

z may be practised in the same way in the strong, weak and intervowel positions.

Exercise 14: Two consonants require especially delicate work in order to articulate and recognize them by lip-reading:

The nasal labial *m*

The nasal dental *n*

They can only be achieved by means of actions which the infant fairly rapidly learns to recognize.

ma is taught by gently placing the lips on the child's hand, somewhat in the manner of kissing. The effect is in direct contrast to the explosive sound of

p and *b*

me mmmmmmmmmmmmmmmmmmmmmmmmmmmmmmmmme

with a fairly prolonged impression of the consonant on the hand of the deaf child. Since the deaf in general are mentally receptive, the sound is imitated. The same procedure should be followed for lip-reading, the lips being lightly pressed together.

Immediate association with the vowels is essential.

mmmmmmmmmmmma mmmmmmmmmmmay   etc.

and in the strong, weak and inter-vowel positions.

In the case of the dental *n*, the teacher clenches his teeth, places his index finger on his own nose and immediately removes it.

The child's finger is placed against the teacher's teeth, so that he appreciates the need for an unemphatic approach to the production of the *n*. The sound sometimes takes a long time to achieve in articulation and lip-reading, but patience and ingenuity can overcome the greatest difficulties.

n should be associated with the vowels in the three positions.

Exercise 15: Articulation and lip-reading of the dentals

d and t

These sounds are relatively easy to acquire. We start with the voiced consonant *d*.

(a) The teacher shows his teeth and gently bites the tip of his tongue.

(b) The syllable *da* must be exploded loudly on to the child's hand. If he is attentive, he will soon imitate the movement of this consonant. The *d* can then be combined immediately with the vowel range

da day dee do doo dwa der dwee

The differentiation of *d* and *t* is rather delicate. The *t* can be exploded more softly against the child's hand than the *d*. If the auditory capacity is there, the process is vastly helped.

The two sounds may be interchanged both for articulation and lip-reading practice:

EXAMPLE: *da day tee do too dwa ter dwee*

Exercise 16: The study of the *ya* sound presents complications since its articulation does not include any external elements. It must, therefore, be associated with other consonants and practised in two parts.

ee............ya

The movement of the hands, sliding across the table, is an excellent aid to bring home the phonetic sound linking the two vowels.

EXAMPLE:

bee............ya
dee............ya etc.

In this field the imagination of the teacher must devise movements capable of stimulating the imitative powers of the child, at the same time as his sensory functions, his manual skill and his motor function in general.

My intention in this work has simply been to describe our timely remedial techniques for the deaf infant. The inestimable advantage of this whole procedure is that the deaf infant, to whom treatment is applied at the age of a few months, acquires the rudiments of speech slightly earlier than the normal child.

Having assessed the ease with which the child has assimilated the phonetic sounds already learnt and the degree to which he has entered into the specialized exercises and acquired correct articulation of the consonants and vowels, taught by means of lipreading and auditory instruction (provided the reanimation of the acoustic nerve allows), the orthophonic teacher may proceed to teach the child to recognize and pronounce words, relating to familiar objects and persons.

For those deaf children who have already passed this early period, Dr. Perdoncini of Nice has designed certain apparatus, which has proved extremely useful for diagnosis and remedial education. I have been able to prove this for myself. I am moreover most grateful to Dr. Perdoncini for his kindness in furnishing for the readers of this book an outline of the principles on which his researches were based, and a description of the design and construction of his apparatus, which offers such obvious benefits to those who are deaf or partially deaf or who are hard of hearing.

Dr. Perdoncini has perfected in his psycho-sensory research laboratory a variety of electronic instruments, designed for use in the diagnosis and remedial education of deaf children.

DIAGNOSIS

The audiometric examination of deaf children is often a very delicate task and subject to errors in measurement.

A special audiometer makes it possible to measure the auditory capacity of very deaf children by means of headphones which transmit the sound impulses. The emission of a continuous tone, as is used in normal audiometry, has proved markedly inferior to the use of a discontinuous tone. The ear rapidly gets used to the continuous tone and the subject is no longer sure whether he can hear anything or not.

Impulse systems, on the other hand, produce an auditory sensation in response to each impulse.

It is clearly necessary that the impulses should be emitted without any transitional stage, otherwise a distortion of the impulses occurs in accordance with an exponential rise and fall. It is moreover easier with this system for the subject to indicate his threshold, since he is asked to record the perception of an auditory sensation by beating time with his hand to the rhythm of the impulses perceived.

This audiometric apparatus is linked to a Peep Show box system fitted with either a powerful loud speaker for binaural investigation of auditory capacity or with channelling of sound to headphones, to allow for assessment of each ear separately. This special audiometer is of use not only for measuring the level of deafness of very deaf children, but can equally be used for all normal audiometric tests, including tests of cochlear function (differential thresholds for frequency, duration and intensity).

REMEDIAL EDUCATION

For purposes of remedial education, deaf children are classified into two groups according to their level of deafness:

(a) *Subjects with a hearing loss of less than 75 dB.* The equipment in use consists essentially of a group of class-rooms fitted with electronic instruments with a system of central amplification and a number of inter-connected individual receivers.

The originality of the concept of these systems, as they are used at the Medical Centres for Phoniatry and Auditory Remedial Education at Villefranche-sur-Mer and La Norville, consists in the fact that it is possible to alter the amplification to suit the auditory curve of the deaf child. Adaptation of amplification to auditory defect is in fact achieved.

(b) *Subjects with a hearing loss greater than 75 dB.* In this case the residual auditory capacity is extremely slight and the subject is not aware of auditory sensations.

It is therefore necessary first of all to establish auditory sensation using sound signals of the most elementary nature.

A "pulsatone" instrument will produce sound impulses, of which the duration, repetition, intensity and frequency (pitch) can be controlled at will. The subject is taught initially to recognize these elementary sounds, then, once auditory sensation has been registered, auditory memory is built up by the progressive acquisition of a succession of sounds, produced by the electronic instrument, and finally of vocal sounds.

Language is built up by a parallel process.

(c) *In all cases of deafness:* An instrument for the kinetic analysis of the voice is used. This is an audio-visual instrument, comprising:

(1) An amplifier of special quality, the amplification curve of which can (on certain apparatus) be exactly adapted to the auditory curve of the subject.

(2) A system of internal summation makes it possible to obtain light discharges (on green and red lamps) the duration of which is proportional to the phonetic groups of the voice. These light discharges are completely automatic and related entirely to the vocal sounds.

A system of filters makes it possible to differentiate between groups of high-pitched and groups of low-pitched phonetic sounds, and between voiced and unvoiced phonemes. The instrument indicates in this way to the deaf subject the number of phonetic sounds in a phrase. They are grouped according to intensity, duration and pitch.

(3) *The appreciation of the rhythm and melody of a phrase:* This instrument may be used not only to give the finishing touches to the voices of those who have received remedial education, but also during the course of, or even at the start of, the remedial treatment, to help the subject to recognize the elementary sounds, represented by impulses.

PARTIALLY DEAF PATIENTS AND THOSE WHO ARE HARD OF HEARING

In addition to the cases of severe deafness there are those children whose acoustic deficiency is less marked, and may even have gone unrecognized, but is none the less a cause of difficulty in relation to the acquisition of language and work at school. These are partially deaf and hard of hearing children.

Under no circumstances should these two categories of children be placed in an Institution for severe cases. They would run the risk of losing the phonetic capital they already possess and of acquiring bad articulatory habits. Nor should they be allowed to attend the so-called "improvement" classes for retarded and backward cases and psychic defectives. The best course is undoubtedly for them to be brought up within the family circle. They should attend school, where their teachers should be asked to seat them in the front row. Surgical or medical treatment may be decisive in these cases.

Special classes do exist where the teacher's voice is amplified by microphone, and diagrams, photographs or instructional films are projected. Unfortunately these are few and bear no relation to the growing number of children who would benefit from them.

As far as we are concerned, the same actions are required of the family as in the case of severely deaf cases. Lip-reading presents no problem, nor does pronunciation.

I have deliberately refrained from referring to the educational drawings and games and all the equipment used for the education of deaf children during the pre-school and school periods. We concern ourselves with these young subjects at an age when there is no possibility of a precise examination. This is the age, I am quite convinced, at which it is vital that attempts should be made to reanimate the acoustic nerve and the auditory organs and muscles. Never again will they be in the same malleable condition. It is vital right from the start to teach them lip-reading and articulation, stage by stage.

Do we want the deaf to speak with a normal, audible voice? Do we want the deaf to articulate correctly? The language used by a deaf person is of the greatest importance. If he can understand, he must also be understood and above all he must pronounce his words correctly and not articulate syllables which are not normally sounded. He must not say, as so many deaf patients who have received education do, *ta bel* for *table* or *ca pi tal* for *capital*.

Do we pay sufficient attention to the speech of the deaf? Hardly, when so many deaf persons, among them the most intelligent, distort their words almost to the point of inaudibility. Do we want the deaf to be able to lip-read fluently all those with whom he comes into contact? Lip-reading is the mainstay of the deaf person, even if a hearing aid gives him some degree of auditory perception.

Do we want the residual auditory capacity of a deaf child (it almost always exists) to be developed to the extent that he can wear a hearing aid, as soon as he is old enough? Deaf children can be fitted with hearing aids at six or seven years old.*

The hearing aid generally amplifies all sounds, which makes the recognition of speech sounds difficult. If the child has already become familiar with syllables, has read and articulated them and can (in the best cases) discriminate between them by ear, he will get the best value out of the hearing aid. In such cases his deafness is improved and he is definitely not mute. This is why I maintain, why I insist that this inappropriate, abusive and humiliating expression "deaf mute" should be definitely erased from our vocabulary. What more dramatic, more false or more agonizing expression can there be for the deaf child or his parents than the term "Asylum for Deaf Mutes"? The impressions it evokes are sorrow, infirmity, exiles on the boundaries of society, and it underlines in its tragic falsity the failure, nay the ignorance, of those whose function it is to save and protect the young.

Will our plea be heard, understood, acted on?

The abolition of a procedure which has become routine, the subject of prejudice, often requires years of patient work. We shall

---

* Indeed at a much earlier age.

have accomplished our task when these unfortunate deaf children return to a normal life in their family and society. This is our most ardent desire. Let it be clearly understood, our aim is not to introduce a new element into the social and school education of children deaf from birth. Our aim is simply to reduce their auditory deficiency and to set them on the road toward education and study. It must never be forgotten that, throughout their school career, the deaf continue to reap the most substantial benefit from auditory training in relation to the normal voice, in spite of the scientific discoveries of the last few years, which have brought indisputable advantages.

It sometimes happens that a child possesses normal auditory perception in its earliest years and then becomes deaf as a result of some encephalopathy or other pathological cause. Sometimes the power of hearing may disappear overnight. If this pathological phenomenon occurs after the child has acquired the power of speech everything possible must be done to preserve it. If the child is sufficiently gifted intellectually, he is able to make use of the storehouse of motor images already present in his brain and, aided by the decisive ability of the brain to replace atrophied function, he may gradually achieve a remarkable virtuosity in the art of deciphering the alphabet of the lips. This is in fact the procedure followed by the normal person, when conversing at a distance. One guesses rather more than one hears.

REMEDIAL EDUCATION

The individual is much less concerned about hearing sounds and noises in general than about "the human voice". For the human ear, the human voice occupies a privileged position. For this reason exercises in auditory discrimination and in auditory and mental attention are of supreme importance.

Exercise 1: First of all practise the syllables which are confused, *p* and *b* for example, or *s* and *z*, *sh* and *zh* (as in pleasure), *d* and *t*; by contrast with the procedure employed for severe cases of deafness, we start immediately with words, including in succession one or other of the syllables which are confused; the child should repeat them immediately.

EXAMPLES: *messy, fill, fool, fussy, sole, Sophy, lace, lost, silence, forest*, etc., *patron, balloon, total, time, deep.* These words should be articulated by the teacher at varying distances from the pupil, making sure that he cannot be seen by the pupil, thus excluding the possibility of lip-reading.

Exercise 2: Articulate a number of "isophonic" syllables, i.e. syllables consisting of sounds identical but for one element.

EXAMPLES: *Toy, boy, coy, joy, rocky, stocky, car, bar, loop, coop, grain, train* etc. Always take care to speak the words at distances appropriate to the auditory capacity of the child.

Exercise 3: Depending on the site of the lesion and the nature of the deafness, sometimes the perception of low-pitched, sometimes of high-pitched sounds is most affected. The orthophonic teacher must establish right from the start which of these categories of sound is least well perceived.

The patient practises with sounds of low and high pitch. They should be grouped according to their range of pitch.

Low pitch: *bomb, renown, sombre, tower, town, Rome, romper,* etc.

High pitch: *taxi, cap, packet, park, misery, discipline,* etc.

Exercise 4: The teacher makes the pupil repeat exactly what he has heard. If the word has been heard incorrectly or not at all, it should be presented in another form, preceding it by a phrase or a couple of words from the same series. Care should be taken, however, not to repeat too often a word which has not been heard, for fear of irritating and disturbing the child.

Exercise 5: Make up phrases of varying length, containing the words that have been heard and reproduced.

EXAMPLES: Mother has taken a taxi.
　　　　　The small boy has taken the cake.
or　　　　My coat is very warm.
or　　　　The floor is very clean.

The teacher should start by articulating these phrases very slowly, gradually working up to normal word speed.

These exercises, I repeat, should be performed at home, out of class hours. The ear of the partially deaf child must be kept in practice by all means possible: conversation (the deaf child should never be isolated), radio, musical practice; reading aloud both by the child and to the child. The worst mistake a deaf person can make is to take refuge in silence and functional inertia.

Inability to hear causes deaf people to lose the habit of listening. This is the danger. The deaf child must play with his normal companions and come into contact with as many people as possible. Outside the remedial periods his deafness should never be alluded to and should be treated as if it did not exist.

There are a large number of poor speakers whose articulation defects, whether of exaggeration or omission, are due to undiagnosed hearing defects, i.e. cases of distorted hearing, not to be regarded as true deafness, but as a modification of the auditory function.

How many children have been blamed by their families for inattentiveness, lack of concentration or even naughtiness, who may have been suffering from the following auditory defects: Distortion of the phonetic pattern as a result of gaps in the auditory field.

Auditory disorientation resulting from disparity or lack of synchronization between the bilateral auditory fields. Retarded auditory perception.

Defective perception of high frequencies only.

All these defects may result in a variety of dysphonias (vocal bi-tonality, functional nasal speech, negative nasality (denasalization), defective or guttural pronunciation) or dyslalias, or sometimes both (absence, substitution or confusion of phonetic sounds.

lisping or impediment in the speech). How very often I have been able to track down a hearing defect of this sort as a basis for a speech defect when the parents had no idea about this slight auditory deficiency. In such case intervention by the laryngologist is necessary and effective.

Apart from this, the methods of auditory education described in this chapter should be employed, suitably adapted to the level of the hearing defect.

Cure the child of his speech defect and stop blaming him for a lack of attention for which he is in no way to blame. On the contrary, he should as far as possible be encouraged and the minimum possible reference made to his auditory defect.

There is no point in preparing a detailed table of remedial education exercises appropriate to the deaf baby. In such cases the teacher must adapt the work to the physical and neural state of the child, the capacity of the mother or person in charge of the child and the very varied whims of a child of a few months. Once deafness has been clearly diagnosed it is best to call in an orthophonic teacher, who is convinced of the necessity of his help for the deaf baby. Let us hope that the followers of this logical and efficient method will become numerous and expert. This is the ultimate purpose of this book.

EXAMPLE OF A REMEDIAL SESSION FOR A YOUNG DEAF CHILD

1. Investigation of residual auditory capacity with attempts to arouse palpebral and oto-cephalogyric reflexes. Note positive and negative responses and the distances at which they occur (5 or 6 times). Carry out the whole procedure twice.

2. Emit vocal sounds very loudly in each ear of the subject

a!............ee..........an etc.

(over a period of 5 minutes).

3. Produce "cascades" of sound for each ear, starting with the appropriate vibrant consonant, coupled with all vowels, at maximum intensity.

rrrrrrrrrrrrrrrrrrrrrrr....a

rrrrrrrrrrrrrrrrrrrrrrr...ay

rrrrrrrrrrrrrrrrrrrrrrrrr....ee

Watch the baby's reactions closely.

This exercise should be practised for a long time, whether the baby responds or not: (at least 30 times in each ear), and if the mother is undertaking the remedial exercises, three times per day.

4. When the child is familiar with the auditory sensation, start exercises combining articulation, auditory function and lip-reading, dealing with one phonetic sound at a time. Do not go on to the next until the sound has been fully mastered: read, pronounced and, though less important, heard.

5. As the child grows up, words and short phrases, relating to everyday life may be treated in the same way. *Daddy, baby, sweet, hullo Mummy, bye-bye Daddy* etc.

For children with severe or partial deafness or who are hard of hearing and who are more advanced, the sequence of the remedial education is the same, although it must be adapted, skilfully and appropriately, to the child's receptivity to education, his psychic and intellectual capital, his talents and his inclinations.

I have tried to bring home to my readers the vital importance of starting the remedial education of the deaf child from the age of seven or eight months. This can be the means of vouchsafing him the power of speech, to which he has a right, and ensuring him a future in relation to family and professional life appropriate to his capabilities, his talents, his inclinations and his own courage. It is nothing less than giving him the opportunity to live like a normal human being.

CHAPTER VI

RETARDED PUPILS

CHILDREN WITH DIFFICULTIES
IN READING, WRITING AND ARITHMETIC.
CHILDREN WITH POOR MEMORY

Included in the category of the mentally defective are those less serious cases who have managed by some means or another to acquire a certain measure of learning. They spend years in the same class and never seem to move to the top. The parents drive them to study harder, while the children sink deeper and deeper into the rut. They fill the school classes without getting any benefit from them. They are a millstone round the neck of the teacher. Remaining at school "on sufferance", these are the backward pupils.

Not without difficulty those who lag behind the rest of the class have learnt to read, to write and to count, but the obstacle of abstraction and reasoning they cannot surmount; that is to say they cannot master mathematics, syntax, analysis, oral discussion which has not been learnt by heart. In some cases their powers of memory are sufficient to allow them to increase their vocabulary, to recite a given text, learn a little history, geography or grammar, thus giving their parents the illusion of progress; but anything requiring thought or judgement is beyond their intellectual capabilities. They cannot grasp the sense of what the teacher is saying; they cannot follow a blackboard demonstration: their powers of attention are defective.

The characteristic feature of their psychological state is slowness which makes every act of intellectual comprehension or elabora-

tion a burden. Admittedly they manage to cope with simple problems, to write short stories, learn and recite their lessons, but
only at the cost of great effort. If questioned about a rule of syntax in relation to a fault in their work, they are incapable of giving
a clear answer; asked to provide a definition of an abstract word
like goodness, justice, heroism, they find themselves in the greatest difficulty; if they are asked to give a number of words relating
to some single subject (e.g. domestic animals, clothes, etc.), they
reveal a surprising poverty in their vocabulary, they apparently
find difficulty in grasping the nature of homonyms, synonyms,
paronyms and antonyms and giving examples of each. They pay
little attention to correct orthography and punctuation. The
shades of meaning, expressed by grammatic agreement, completely
escape them. In grammar, syntax, mathematics and composition,
they wallow in the mire. If their powers of memory permit them to
rise above the level of their mediocre capacity, they recite confi-
dently their history, geography or foreign language lessons, provided a sudden question is not interjected to upset the order of the
work they have prepared. How often have La Fontaine's delightful fables, so fresh, so full of common sense and wisdom, with
their pictures taken straight from life, been trodden underfoot by
iconoclasts, who could not recognize their virtues. Those gentle
harmonies of Racine, what rude shocks have been administered to
their winged rhythms, as unfortunate pupils stumble over their
subtle cadences.

These misusers and abusers of the works of the great are not
much given to conversation. The questions of their families are
parried with short phrases. If by any chance they have any command of language, they fill their speech with stereotyped phrases,
poorly linked together, and generally irrelevant. Very often their
delivery is irregular, they stumble over consonants or whole words,
and articulate badly. If they can read, they read slowly; they suffer
from bradylexia.

Even at play, these backward pupils do not behave like normal
children of their age. Their games lack life, they cannot snatch the
opportunity of a catch, nor leap forward quickly nor jump skil-

fully. Their motor functions too are slow, their movements poorly co-ordinated.

They will never escape from this impasse, unless they are sent to some source which provides remedial education or individual tuition from qualified personnel. They should also be given the appropriate medical treatment, especially hormone therapy, to accelerate their intellectual and motor functions. We should not set our sights too high; our only aim is to give these unfortunate psycho-motor defectives the opportunity of shaking off the stifling inertia that holds them in thrall and of enabling them to make their own living. These children are in fact the marginal cases between true mental defectives, described above, and those children who do not fall below the lower level of normal intelligence.

The backward pupil has been, and continues to be, the subject of study and research; numerous works have been, are being and will be devoted to these backward pupils. Their case is tragic, no one can fail to appreciate that the long-standing deficit in the recruitment of teachers coupled with the steady increase of children of school age, has given rise to a situation in which children, presenting special difficulty in regard to teaching, are as good as lost.

These unfortunate children are lost amongst the great mass of their companions. They are not always intellectually retarded, far from it, but they are slow to understand, slow to assimilate, slow to think and slow to work. Learning to read presents great difficulty to them; they may be described as "bradylexics" or "dyslexics" and "dysorthographics", they are slow in their psychic and motor function. Their inner life is often lived intensely, but their fetters bind them so securely that they are thought to be indifferent and idle, whereas in fact they are frustrated, maladapted, humiliated, hurt and unhappy. In the family circle the reassurance given by a compliment or an approving word is unknown to them. Bad at arithmetic, with poor powers of memory they struggle to learn their lessons, and recite them badly. Anyway they are rarely asked to do so. The teachers have no time to give them the care they require. Experts in holding down the bottom places in the class, they are prisoners of their own surrender to life and have given up all hope of rising again. Have we not heard them called "cretins"?!

When the time comes for examinations, failure is certain.

All this is deplorable. These children, who are unsuited for group instruction, can make real progress with individual tuition when they can learn to concentrate their attention, develop their powers of imagination, understanding and memory. Their intelligence, which was withering away in chains, is awakened and set free. Reading and writing are mastered, arithmetic seems less formidable, powers of memory are developed.

At the present time efforts are being made to provide special education for dyslexic and backward pupils of all types. These children require specialist and psychological teaching. Visual and psychological instructional aids have been produced for them. Medical treatment can be of great value in effecting improvements in their condition. My only aim in this field is to enumerate a number of exercises which have proved of great assistance to certain backward pupils whom I have treated, enabling them to "go up in class".

1. This exercise is based on the effect which the acquisition of rhythm has on cerebral activity. Make the pupil with outstretched hands beat time with two, three, four, five and six beats in a bar. This must be practised with absolute precision and energy.

In time with this the pupil reads off a slate (I have already pointed out that subjects with defective vision did not take part in our work) all the consonants and vowels.

The easier measures of time, two, three and four are chosen initially.

The consonants:

b–k–d–f–g–zh–sh–l–m–n–p–r–s–t–v–ks–y–z.

The pupil should then recite them by heart in groups of four, from the first to the fourth, then the fourth to the first.

EXAMPLE: *be–ke–de–fe* in 4-time, 15 times   *each group*

        fe–de–ke–be

2. The same exercise with all the vowel sounds, which are read aloud clearly: *a* (p*a*t)–*e* (p*e*t)–*ay* (p*a*y)–*air–er–ee–y–o* (p*o*t)–*or–oh* (g*o*ld)–*oo–wa–wee*.

Add the consonant *f*, which may also be written *ph*.

When this exercise has been completed, the pupil should read all the syllables.

EXAMPLES: *coo coo–chap–jay–lot–man–men–pan–cur*, etc. Not more than five minutes at a time.

3. When the child starts to get familiar with the various vowels, consonants and groupings, show him orally, with the aid of lip-reading if necessary, the letters which form the beginning of mono-syllabic words.

EXAMPLES: *ball, salt, pat, toy, let, milk, rain, note, sole, town,* etc.

4. The words listed above should be learnt by heart, then spelt, first *forwards*, then *backwards*. The results of this exercise can be rapid and decisive. At least twenty words per day should be spelt out in this way at home.

EXAMPLE: Spell the word *page*, beating out the letters in four time with both hands.

page	the numbers of letters being spelt out do not always fit in with the
then	time. This is not important. One beat of four is left unfinished or
e g a p	an extra one is begun. The important thing is to maintain the
1–2–3–4	rhythm.

This exercise is extremely valuable for normal adolescents with infinite variations. It is worth noting that backward pupils suffering from some psychic deficiency have a greater facility for spelling backwards than forwards. Normal subjects, on the other hand, find this operation very hard. I have treated both primary school pupils and students from higher classes in this way and obtained positive results.

The words must of course become progressively longer and more difficult. Where an adolescent is being treated, the choice of words should be guided by his subjects of study or intended profession.

5. Exercise for powers of memory, co-ordination and adaptation to school lessons. The nine movements given below should be executed *by heart* (standing upright):

(1) Raise the right arm above the head.

(2) Stretch it out horizontally.

(3) Raise the right leg and bend the knee.

(4) Tap out one beat on the floor energetically.

(5) Stretch out the left arm horizontally.

(6) Raise the left arm above the head.

(7) Raise the left leg and bend the knee.

(8) Tap out one beat on the floor energetically.

(9) Lower both arms, one from above the head, the other from the horizontal position.

6. In time with these movements, one word per movement, recite *by heart* from the first to the ninth, then from the ninth to the first, the following words:

noun, article, adjective, pronoun, verb, adverb, preposition, conjunction, interjection. The whole exercise to be practised nine times.

7. Spell these nine words by heart, forwards and backwards.

8. Carry out the following movements:

(1) Bend the knees (stretching them wide astride) and extend the arms horizontally forwards.

(2) Extend the right leg.

(3) Return it to the original position.

(4) Extend the left leg.

(5) Return it to the original position.

(6) Raise the arms above the head.

(7) Rise to the upright position and lower the arms.

9. In time with these movements, articulate the fourteen signs of punctuation:

Full stop	.	Articulate these words to a beat of 7, in time
Comma	,	with the movements given above. The
Colon	:	movements will be run through twice to
Semi-colon	;	cover the fourteen signs of punctuation

Dieresis	··
Apostrophe	'
Open bracket	(
Close bracket	)
Open inverted commas	"
Close inverted commas	"
Hyphen	-
Interrogation mark	?
Exclamation mark	!
Ellipse	...

10. Spell all the above words backwards and forwards: this is not always easy.

11. Make the pupil compose short dictation exercises. Start with short phrases, built round a word furnished by the teacher.

EXAMPLES: *forest, walk, cape, golf, grammar, verb, beach, blackboard.*

The pupil composes a phrase on the basis of these words. The teacher notes it — or remembers it. When all eight phrases are complete, they are dictated back to the pupil, who subsequently carries out a grammatical analysis of each phrase, pointing out the place of each word in the phrase.

EXAMPLE: These deep forests cover an immense area.

The pupil should then parse each word, giving part of speech, whether singular or plural, type of adjective etc., and spell all the words forwards and backwards. These exercises are similar to scholastic exercises. We point this out simply to emphasize the difference between remedial education and normal scholastic work.

EXERCISES FOR PUPILS WEAK AT ARITHMETIC

1. Sitting down with hands outstretched on the table.

Close the hands
Open the hands
Separate the fingers
Bring them together again.

Perfect synchronization in the movements of the fingers *must* be achieved.

2. To a beat of 4, count at the rate of one numeral per beat from 1 to 10, then to 20 and back to 1. Carry on in groups of 20, i.e. 20 to 40, 40 to 60, etc. up to 100.

All the time it is important to count upwards and downwards.

3. Pronounce forwards and backwards the two-digit numbers.

EXAMPLE: 75———7–5, 5–7

4. Standing up:

(a) Join the hands
(b) Move the right arm sideways
(c) Move the left arm sideways
(d) Stretch one leg forwards
(e) Bend the knee
(f) Strike the ground with the foot

5. In time with these movements, rhythmically executed, pronounce forwards and backwards three-digit numbers (from the first figure to the third and from the third figure to the first). The teacher provides the numbers if the pupil cannot do so.

EXAMPLE: 325

Repeat in time with the movements, having learnt by heart:

   3–2–5
   5–2–3

This exercise should be practised ten times each day.

6. Thirdly add the figures cumulatively, still in time.

EXAMPLE: 3 and 2 is 5 and 5 is 10.

7. Numbers containing 4, 5 and 6 digits are treated in the same way, the teacher giving exercises involving dissociated movements to fit in with the number of digits.

Example of movements for 6 digits: upright position:

Count out a beat of three with the right hand only.

In the same rhythm, strike the left thigh with the left hand 3 times vigorously.

Beat out 3 taps on the floor with the left foot.

Beat out 3 taps on the floor with the right foot.

This exercise must of course be practised on its own first, then articulating the digits forwards and backwards and finally adding them. These exercises, which are designed to stimulate cerebral activity, can be extremely effective, provided they are given and performed energetically. The teacher should give the pupil an example of what is required and go through the movements with him.

8. An effective exercise for pupils weak in arithmetic, is to count, to a given beat, the even numbers in a given range, upwards and downwards, then in the same way the odd numbers.

9. It is a good idea, if possible, to dictate at each period the numbers which the pupil finds difficult to recognize. There is often confusion between 4 and 7, 9 and 6, 2 and 3.

10. There is a great deal of equipment available for the education of those who find it difficult to count, notably that produced by Louis Colle (Monte Carlo and Alpes-Maritimes). In my view the abacus which he has designed seems based on logic and sound teaching principles. It has already proved itself.

The treatment for the child weak in arithmetic can be extended to cover concrete exercises and written work. The treatment I have described has but one single aim: to develop, by means of psycho-neural co-ordination, the cerebral and intellectual possibilities of the backward pupil. This in turn stimulates the function of the cerebro-motor mechanisms and creates a spirit of compliance and comprehension which makes the child more accessible to normal school methods.

The use of multiplication tables, as they are normally taught at school, should be avoided. The children recite them automatically, using mnemonic connections, without thinking them out. This is all right for normal, but not for backward pupils.

For backward pupils they may be mastered in the following way:

> 6 times 1 is 6
> 1 times 6 is 6
> 2 times 6 is 12
> 6 times 2 is 12

all the way up to 6 times 12 is 72, and 12 times 6 is 72. Then come down again from 12 to 1.

ABACUS DESIGNED AT THE CENTRE FOR REMEDIAL EDUCATION, MONTE CARLO

(Director: Louis Colle)

It is a vertical abacus with freely-mounted beads in the shape of a rectangular plate, divided longitudinally into three sections. The two outer parts are in the form of cups, designed to receive the beads, which are removed from the pins. On the inner section are mounted two rows of pins, on to which the beads are threaded. The first row contains ten pins of unequal lengths, each capable of holding between 1 and 10 beads, but no more than the given number. A stud, on to which no beads can be threaded, represents zero. In front of each pin is a square showing the colour and number of beads which the pin is capable of taking (between 1 and 10). The second row of pins, on the other hand, are all of the same length and can take 10 beads exactly. As in the case of the first row, a coloured square shows the colour and number of beads, which each pin can take (by tens, 10, 20, 30 etc. up to 100). Finally a separate pin, holding 9 beads, is used only for "Carry-over" figures.

It is easy to see that an abacus of this type can teach at the same time the figure, the number and the colour, using the first row of pins. By proper use of both rows, however, it is possible to teach the child addition and subtraction (with or without "Carry-over" figures) as well as multiplication and division up to 100.

This abacus is at present in use at the Centre for Remedial Education at Monte Carlo where positive results have been obtained with backward pupils and those who are weak in arithmetic. It also helps in explaining the four basic operations of arithmetic.

CHAPTER VII

PSYCHO-NEURAL MOTOR DEFECTS

TONIC, CLONIC AND COMBINED TONIC-CLONIC STAMMERING, DISORDERED RHYTHM, STUTTERING AND PSEUDO-NORMALITY

I am putting at the head of this chapter the principle laid down by the late lamented Dr. Gérard de Parrel: "The governing factor in regard to the recovery of children whose faculties are for whatever reason impaired, is early treatment". Despite the truth of this advice, this instruction is neglected by the world of families, doctors, nurses and social workers. For months and years they wait for an improvement which does not manifest itself, in spite of the most varied medical treatment. The defect grows with the child. The child with his psycho-neural motor defect becomes progressively an invalid, a "complete invalid" and a martyr to his affliction.

Adult stutterers are in fact real invalids. One must have been brought into contact with them professionally to know the measure of their despair. If those who are disabled were grouped as more fortunate and less fortunate, these people would be counted among the most unfortunate, since no one has any sympathy for them and some even make fun of them. Many legitimate human aspirations are not for them; their disability bars the way. Whether in the family, at school or in society, they continually come up against the same obstacles. They are everywhere in a state of anxiety, if not in the grip of anguish and phobia. The largeness of their numbers makes them even more deserving of the attention of the remedial worker. According to published statistics, they account for some 1 per cent of the total child population; boys predominate amongst them (three boys to one girl).

The stammer is a psycho-neural motor co-ordination syndrome, the predominant manifestation of which is a spasmodic respiratory-phonetic dysfunction. The onset is generally in childhood, very often simultaneously with the acquisition of speech — always against a background of emotional and affective instability and weakness of the neuro-glandular systems. Stammering is not, strictly speaking, a speech disability, since, under certain conditions, articulation and delivery may become normal, and it could be said, on the other hand, that some subjects stammer with their hands and feet. It is a complex functional disorder, which takes the form of a disorganization of the co-ordinated process of elocution. This respiratory-phonetic disorder is characterized by a series of spasmodic movements, occurring at irregular intervals under the influence of badly co-ordinated psychic stimulation. The spasm is the functional signature of this disability and emotional dysfunction its underlying cause. In reality it is a co-ordination neurosis; the variability of the manifestations of the disorder provides the proof of the predominance of psychic influences.

Stammering is manifested in disturbances of the tonus and of muscular co-ordination, sometimes generalized, sometimes localized in the respiratory and speech organs. There are subjects who — as I have observed — stammer not only with their speech organs, but with their hands and feet. I have treated stammering subjects who if brought into contact with another person, could not even shake them by the hand, or take a pen to write, even for the purpose of signing their name. They were in a state of total inhibition, but their delivery was normal. They were suffering in effect from graphic and gestural stammering. In brief, from the motor point of view, these sufferers from a lack of co-ordination are, in a mild form, asynergics, dystonics and dysmetrics; in the majority of cases they are left-handed. The further back one goes, the clearer it becomes that all the implements which men have used, to defend themselves, to attack, to build, to till the soil or produce food, have been designed for right-handed persons. "The dominance of the one hemisphere over the other is essential, in order to ensure the correct performance of bilateral acts especially of speech", wrote Ombredane, "Stammering is the result of failure to achieve a unified control, of the failure of the one hemisphere to dominate the other".

If a left-handed child starts to stammer, one must avoid trying to alter his motor habits, since this would be running directly counter to the required aim. Left-handedness is a simple constitutional factor and one should therefore not try to reverse it. Do we ask the right-handed person to become left-handed?

The right or left-handed orientation of the child is often unknown to his immediate family. The mother, burdened with the cares of family and home, has not the leisure to observe carefully the particular motor characteristics of her children, especially if she has several. At the first interview with mother and child, I have often observed and remarked on the fact that the child is left-handed (using the left hand to shake hands or to pick something up) and heard the mother reply, "I don't know... I never noticed anything... he eats with his right-hand"... but the child is ambidextrous and therefore similar to a left-handed child. How often have I heard the mother or person responsible for the stammering child say, with stupid naïveté, "Give Madame your right hand" or, in the popular idiom, "your 'good' hand". It is all one can do to force an admission that, at the motor level, both hands are equal and the standards of aesthetic judgement, good manners and education cannot be made to apply to them.

A true stammer, a childhood stammer, may not manifest itself simultaneously with the acquisition of speech. It may be set off by some psychic trauma or sudden fear: a family scene, an accident, a forceful reproach or punishment. During the era of the bombing 1940 to 1945, many psycho-motor disorders were the result of terror, though not so many as one might have supposed, since in this case the traumatic shock had been sustained collectively. The terror reflex must act on the psychic and nervous centres of the child as an individual.

In practice a background of hypersensitivity and hyperdevelopment of the motor function in the young child prepares the way for the pathological outcome of a violent experience. A normal person, subjected to the same emotional shock, would not suffer the same pathological reaction. Some cases of stammering are related to serious disturbances of the personality or the affective centre and are brought on by conflict. In such cases psycho-therapy is essential. It is thus clear that the term multisensory remedial education is entirely appropriate, since the wide variety of the treatment applied is exactly suited to the wide variety of psycho-neural motor disorders from which the subject suffers.

Some dysphasic patients suffer from a singular defect, which may lead the uninitiated observer to imagine that it is a special form of stammering. Such is the case of children who repeat spontaneously and almost incorrigibly one or more words or a short phrase. They are suffering from "palilalia". Whereas the stammering subject says, "A bbbeautiful bbbboat", the palilalic subject will say, "A beautiful boat, a beautiful boat ..." *ad nauseam*, but without any trace of impediment, hesitation or syllabic confusion. This disorder belongs unfortunately to the class of those of encephalopathic origin. Some patients are found to suffer from "echolalia", the symptom of which is to repeat a phrase spoken by the teacher or by his parents. If, for example, such defectives are given a simple order, "Lift your arms", they will repeat several times, "Lift your arms, lift your arms". Such speech disorders have nothing in common with stammering and should not be confused with it.

There are two forms of stammering: tonic and clonic. The characteristic feature of the first type is a relatively stable contraction of the muscles responsible for the emission and articulation of speech; the speech organs contract into a cramped attitude, especially if the initial syllable begins with an occlusive voiced consonant: *be–de–ge*; or unvoiced: *pe–te–ke*. If the initial syllable begins with a vowel, a parasitic initial occlusive consonant may be superimposed. The state of tension is so marked that it seems impossible for the syllable to be articulated, then the spasm passes abruptly and the syllable explodes.

In clonic stammering, on the other hand, the syllables, especially the initial syllables are repeated convulsively as a result of a series of subintrant muscular contractions. The tonic stammerer will say "L...l...lazy B...b...bones", while the clonic stammerer will say "La...la...lazy Bo...bo...bones".

Tonic stammering is often complicated by generalized contractions, the subject moves his hands with frenzy, stamps on the floor with his feet, throws his head back and gives the impression of unco-ordinated agitation. All trace of synchronized movement disappears, in relation not only to delivery, articulation and respiration, but also to movements of the head and trunk. Clonic stammering is more limited in the repercussions on motor function and movement.

For some time now research has been carried out on the radio-cinematic study of the mechanism of speech. It has been discovered that tonic and clonic stammering are physiologically and pathologically distinct phenomena. This will open new horizons in the study of these two disorders. From the psychological point of view, subjects suffering from these two types of stammering present very different personality characteristics. Even amongst children, the former are severely inhibited, tormented, anguished, but often intelligent, while the latter are less affected by their disability and are often irritating, especially to others. As far as they are themselves concerned, they reveal a benign form of this infirmity. In some subjects the two forms are mixed, which in addition goes to prove that the two forms can exist together in the same person. Tension and repetition occur; this is the tonic-clonic stammer.

Since this work is devoted to the description of multisensory remedial treatment, it seems to me appropriate to adapt similar remedial techniques to these two disabilities. This conforms to our principle of providing treatment "to measure", for complex phonation, speech and psycho-neural motor defects.

Stammering is a functional complex, the characteristic features of which are confusion and an insufficiency of speech movements. A torrent of consonants, an inaudible delivery, a marked lack of rhythm and an absence of co-ordinated articulation. In general those who suffer from this disorder are hypotonic and have faulty respiration. For the greater part of the time they are practically normal and the function of their cerebral motor centres is in no way defective.

REMEDIAL TREATMENT
FOR STAMMERING AND STUTTERING

These two disorders are given similar remedial treatment, the only difference being that the multiple symptoms of the stammerer are more impressive than those of the stutterer. They take longer to correct and exhibit greater complexity in their duration and in the type of methods required, but the same general principles of remedial education apply to both disorders.

In treatment of this sort, remedial teachers must regard themselves as craftsmen working on the repair of human material, in other words the work is hard and painful. The first step is to gain the confidence of the child, learn how to calm him, amuse him, make him feel he wants to come to the remedial sessions. The teacher must become the "friend" of his pupil, retaining at the same time his authority and prestige.

Teachers, specializing in this type of neuro-psycho-motor education, must possess, as I indicated at the beginning of this book, a complex of qualities and gifts, which are not always found in the same person; physical stamina, vocal intensity, even respiration, muscular suppleness, good sight, good hearing, straightforward and friendly appearance, eloquence, faultless articulation and a resonant voice. I crave indulgence for my insistence on this point; the results of the application of this effective and many sided form of remedial education can be so successful if the teacher is worthy of his task, that I cannot impress too strongly on those who wish to undertake this work, that EVERYTHING DEPENDS on the teacher and the trouble he takes.

One must have the "sacred fire of devotion", in order to adopt a profession of this sort. It is none the less the finest of all professions, it demands love for the suffering child, the passionate desire to cure him and complete forgetfulness of self.

The teacher will, moreover, himself experience a sort of a rebirth, a physical and psychic enrichment of the self. He is a universal donor of energy, in the same way as there are donors of blood. Of his own free-will and with dynamic initiative he supplies transfusions of energy.

There is moreover the important question of a psychic emanation from the teacher to the pupil, a real psychic affinity must be created between them. That is why I appeal to the physical and moral integrity of the individual. None of his reactions, his gifts, his possibilities, his faults and his defects must remain hidden. In the course of many professional visits in Europe, during many consultations I have held for remedial education, I have noticed the inadequacy of the techniques employed. In regard to stammering in particular the absence of a technique of wide application is very sorely felt. We are dealing here with such a complex system of spasmodic disorders, inhibition, lack of co-ordination and disturbances of rhythm and equilibrium that a course of remedial education, dealing only with the aspect of phonetics and rhythm, must run the risk of being ineffective. The stammer is only a symptom of a psycho-cerebral motor syndrome. The patient must be made to undertake physical, psychic, cerebral and phonetic exercises.

RESPIRATORY EDUCATION

1. We start with respiratory training, using the "spirometer". We use the "Plent Respirator", which is particularly suited for this type of training. Since the water is coloured pink and a glass flask is used, the child can watch the course of his own respiration, which is a good means of control. The instrument incorporates "end-pieces", designed for respiration through the mouth and nose. Inspiration should be carried out silently and quickly, while expiration should be long-drawn-out. The respirator is so designed

that it can be set and adapted to the strength and resistance of the child under treatment. The child is placed sitting, very upright, on a stool in front of the table on which the instrument has been placed, with the elbows to the sides and the head straight. Practise for a quarter of an hour, preferably twice a day. The operation of nasal respiration is a little more delicate. Children with a nasal obstruction (slight deformation of the tissue, hypertrophy of a nasal septum) find it difficult initially to breathe through the nose. In such cases one nostril should be deliberately obstructed, while the child breathes through the other. The nasal expiration should also, of course, be as long-drawn-out as possible. Four to five minutes training for each nostril. Care must be taken to ensure that during respiration through the mouth, the child keeps his lips tight up against the mouth-piece. Sustained gripping with the lips is a good exercise in directed action.

The duration of expiration plays an important part in the technique of remedial education. These "pneumokinetic" exercises foster suppleness in the movements of the diaphragm and exercise a secondary effect on the neuro-vegetative system by this stimulation of the diaphragm.

2. The pupil should be expected to meet two particular requirements: To attend all remedial sessions punctually and properly turned out, with hair brushed and hands clean.

When dealing, as we are with a social class that attends hospitals and dispensaries, one cannot expect elegance; the pupil can, however, be expected to present himself for the remedial session properly turned out, out of respect for the teacher. How many young children have acquired a better standard of behaviour as a result of the attentions and cautionary words of the teacher! Even amongst the better off, I have seen improvements and amongst the mothers too.

Great care is needed, however; some pupils, both boys and girls, are, by contrast, too wrapped up in themselves. They are vain, coquettish and selfish. It is worth while struggling against this excessive refinement, which is found, strangely enough, in combination with a neglect of the most elementary rules of cleanliness. The teacher must use his influence to re-establish the balance and strike the happy mean.

Respiratory training should as far as possible be carried out at home leaving the lesson period free for the important process of analysing the exercises to be performed, since it is while adapting his cerebral commands to the performance of co-ordination exercises that the stammering subject makes the greatest progress. This underlines the importance of devising original exercises for each period. Once motor automatism has been acquired, the practising of dissociated movements is less effective.

It must be emphasized that the basic exercises (maxilla, lips, tongue, naso-labial groove, angles of the lips and violent clearing of the throat — 100 times per day) should never be omitted. "Twice a day at home". During the lesson period the teacher should check the manner in which the exercises have been carried out at home, to see whether they have been performed energetically with deliberation and precision.

If the child who stammers suffers also, for some undetectable reason, from dysphonia or dyslalia, omits or confuses his consonants or alters the timbre of his vowels, these defects must be corrected first. Sometimes they are found in combination.

For the necessary methods of correction, reference should be made to the chapters devoted to dysphonias, dyslalias and defects of speech and language. Bear in mind also "tics", choreic movements of the face, neck, limbs and dorsal muscles; watch for them and treat them with the appropriate rhythmic exercises.

When all this has been performed and checked (when repairing a machine, does not one check all the parts?) we can begin the psycho-neural co-ordination exercises.

PRACTICAL EXERCISES IN THE SITTING POSITION

Exercise 1: To be practised after the basic exercises. Seal the lips hermetically (so that the mucous membrane cannot be seen).

Clench the teeth (they should remain clenched throughout the exercise).

In one sharp movement, open wide the lips, revealing both rows of teeth, then seal them together again (40 times per day, preferably in two sessions).

Exercise 2: Inflate the cheeks with the lips pressed together. In time with the second beat, hollow the cheeks, then inflate them again (40 times).

Those with motor defects and some who stammer often find the greatest difficulty in blowing out their cheeks. It is in any case a very useful little test. By patience and mimicry it can be achieved. One must always persevere, never allow a pupil to become discouraged, but indefatigably practise the movement in front of him and with him.

Exercise 3: I suggest that teachers should be careful not to leave around objects capable of distracting the pupil's attention, such as, for example, mirrors in which he will never tire of watching himself. The teacher should avoid wearing jewels, bracelets, rings or brooches which always fascinate children.

Close the eyes firmly (so that the eyelashes hardly show), then open them sharply, raising the eyebrows and forehead muscles as if in an expression of great astonishment.

The teacher then orders:

Raise (the eyebrows), close etc. (30 times).

Exercise 4: Combine exercises 1 and 3 in the following way (if the child is able to do so):

(a) Close the lips tightly over the clenched teeth, at the same time opening wide the eyes, raising the eyebrows and muscles of the forehead.

(b) Close the eyes completely, opening wide the lips over the clenched teeth and vice versa (20 times in succession).

Practise these dissociated movements of the muscles and face. This is in fact an exercise to dissociate synchronized movements and must be carried out rhythmically. It takes a fairly long time to achieve perfectly. The teacher practises the exercise, of course, with the pupil.

Very few stammering subjects, children or adults, can beat time correctly. If they happen to have practised scales, they beat time weakly, without energy or precision. They have to be taught to hold the hand stiff with the index finger pressed against the thumb. The hands then become stiff as little sticks. Always practise both hands, in order to give left-handed subjects the opportunity to use their right hands, and right-handed subjects the chance to practise with the left hand as well as with the right.

Point out that it is better to beat time not with the whole arm, but with the upper arm pressed tightly against the body. In this way we avoid the wide sweeping gestures to which arhythmics are addicted.

When this has been done, start to beat time in bars of two beats, on the orders "knees" and "shoulders", given by the teacher. The pupil strikes his knees (without letting his hands rebound) with the hands sideways, then strikes his shoulders. Take particular care that the second beat is not too high (behind the ears) or too low (on the upper arms); the shoulder must be struck directly and with precision. Teach the pupil to stress the first beat or strong beat, the central pillar of the rhythm (in this instance the beat coincides with the striking of the knees).

I have deliberately refrained from using the metronome or piano to mark the rhythm of my remedial exercises. It is essential that the subject should incline his own will-power, his cerebral faculties, his nervous system, even his whole self toward the rhythm. To adapt the prescribed dissociated movements to the relatively precise rhythm of a metronome or a musical beat is not enough to create and develop the "inner rhythm". The lesser effort brings a lesser reward. It is the task of the teacher to instil into his pupils the attitude and the rhythmic movement, which leads to beneficial training.

Exercise 5: To a beat of two, strictly maintained:

(a) push the lips well forward without letting them touch,
(b) open them as wide as possible. This is designed to exercise the orbicular muscles of the lips and the cheek muscles.

It bears comparison with the exercises *oo* and *ee*, but on a larger scale. It is carried out in silence.

Exercise 6: To a beat of two:

(a) Make a loud sound with the mouth closed.
(b) Then immediately produce the two labial consonants.

pe be

both to be enunciated on the second beat, going over from the position for the loud sound with the mouth closed to the production of *pe* without opening the mouth at all (20 times morning and evening).

Exercise 7: Still to a beat of two, articulate and learn by heart the series of phonetic consonants and vowels which will subsequently be employed in numerous exercises practised in the upright position:

ba, *bay*, *bee*, *bo*, *boo*, *bwa*, *ber*, at the rate of one syllable per beat.

The same series of vowels should then be articulated with all the other consonants:

k d f g j sh l m n p r s t v x(ks) y z

Practise every day from the first to the eighteenth and from the eighteenth to the first (by heart).

Exercise 8: Teach the pupil to practise the following movements to a beat of three:

1	2	3
Strike the knees	Stretch the arms sideways	Strike the shoulders

with emphasis on the first beat and energetic sideways stretching of the arms.

In time with the beat of three:

Clear the throat, followed by:

articulation of *ka!*   energetic articulation and
articulation of *gan!*   very resonant voice

(30 times morning and evening).

Exercise 9: With the lips together, but not pressed tightly, move the labial block in all directions energetically (like a rabbit eating a carrot).

This is a difficult exercise. One minute per day.

During this exercise the hands may carry out at eye level the puppet-show movements.

Exercise 10: (a) With fingers stretched out straight, count out a beat of four with both hands:

1	2	3	4
Strike the knees	Cross the hands on the chest	Stretch the arms sideways	Strike the shoulders

(b) The following exercise for the maxilla, lips and tongue in time with the beat:

(1) Open the mouth sharply (lower the maxilla right down).
(2) Put out the tongue bringing it to a point.
(3) Draw in the tongue without closing the mouth.
(4) Close the mouth.

All exactly in time with the beat. A point to note is that pupils are always inclined to close the mouth at the same time as they draw in the tongue. They must be made to carry out the four movements separately which is an excellent exercise in co-ordination.

Exercise 11: Move the tongue round the inside of the mouth at top speed. Lips and cheeks should be moved also. Produce sound during this exercise.

Exercise in "undifferentiated articulation" which we term "stuttering".

This exercise can be carried out even by small children. At the start it can be practised without sound in order to familiarize the movements. Subsequently it is practised aloud.

Exercise 12: Practise the previous exercise in conjunction with the puppet-show hand movements at eye level; the hands are rotated rapidly on the wrists; an extremely rapid movement is essential.

The teacher in charge of these combined exercises himself counts one! two! in exact time and in a loud voice (20 times at least morning and evening).

Exercise 13: The same exercise as "stuttering" (Ex. 11), undifferentiated articulation, associated with the following movements: rotation at full speed of the hands one above the other at chest height, with the arms outstretched.

This exercise must be practised with the hands as far as possible away from the body. With young children I call it the "squirrel in the cage" exercise, the movements of the hands being reminiscent of those of the squirrel's paws on a roller.

The puppet gestures may for example be continued for ten bars of 2-time, then an abrupt change to the "squirrel in the cage" for ten bars, followed by the puppet-gestures once again. The alternation of these exercises on the orders of the teacher provides good training in attention and rhythm.

Exercise 14: The child sits down in front of a table, with hands on the table, and lifts one hand after the other, lifting at the same time the fingers of both hands and bringing them down to strike the table. Starting with the thumbs, play imitation five-note scales (up and down).

Thumb	Index finger	2nd	3rd	4th finger
1	2	3	4	5

and down again; 4th, 3rd, 2nd, index finger and thumb.

In time with these movements the child articulates short phrases, one syllable per beat:

"I learn to read and then to write"
"I can ar ti cu late better now".

This exercise is extremely effective and can be practised in everyday life, so that the child can learn to speak slowly with even rhythmic syllables. If the child knows how to read, he can be made to read aloud, pronouncing the syllables in time with movements of the fingers. Using this exercise, the child may be made to give the names of the fingers, given above. They should be recited by heart from the first to the fifth and the fifth to the first.

Exercise 15: As soon as the child has learnt to beat out bars of 2, 3 and 4 time, he should be taught to beat out bars of 5 and 6 time:

1	2	3	4
Strike the knees	Stretch the arms sideways	Strike the shoulders	Strike the knees

5

Strike the shoulders

Beats 1 and 4 should be stressed, both in movement and voice, although their proper time value should be observed. The child must be able to count aloud from 1 to 5 and 5 to 1.

Bars of six time

This can be practised in two ways:
Either two consecutive bars of 3 or a more frequent procedure:

1	2	3
Strike the knees	Strike the knees	Strike the knees
4	5	6
Strike the shoulders	Strike the shoulders	Strike the shoulders

(strike the shoulders exactly, not up toward the ears, as children are inclined to do).

Exercise 16: Still in the sitting position, the child reaches the stage of being able to go in succession through bars of 3, 4, 5 and 6 time, counting at the same time: one! two! one! two! three! one! two! three! four! for each separate bar, making sure to start each bar with an emphatic one.

It is a good thing to do this exercise the other way round, i.e. starting with the 6 beat bar. Count in the same way: six! five! four! three! two! one! etc. down to two! one! for the two-beat bar.

Children with a stammer find this last exercise difficult to master. The first part only may be used in appropriate cases.

Exercise 17: In exactly the same way six syllable phrases are articulated in time, the stress coming always on the first syllable: Examples of suitable words:

> telephone exchanges
> Highland lads and lasses
> terrapin and tortoise

Practise as follows:

2-time	High	land				
3-time	High	land	lads			
4-time	High	land	lads	and		
5-time	High	land	lads	and	lass	
6-time	High	land	lads	and	lass	es

If the child can do it, practise in the reverse order:

6-time	es	lass	and	lads	land	High
5-time		lass	and	lads	land	High
4-time			and	lads	land	High
3-time				lads	land	High
2-time					land	High

This is a hard exercise, but it develops judgement, rhythm, memory and articulation. Other phrases should be treated in the same way.

EXERCISES IN THE UPRIGHT POSITION

Principal psycho-neural co-ordination exercises

Just as in earlier times a skilful coachman was able to drive three, four, five or six horses, taking account of the individual characters and reactions of each, in the same way our young pupils, suffering from multiple disorders, must learn to exercise simultaneous control over their thoughts, their speech, the movements of their hands, and of their feet, subjecting all these to the control of the will in accordance with an exact rhythm. This is why we practise the simultaneous performance of dissociated movements. Those amenable to such methods are for the most part incapable of keeping more than one idea in their head at once ... With them a short-circuit is formed between the thought and its expression: the spoken word.

Speech, however, is movement. These subjects often find it impossible to co-ordinate the processes of speaking and walking. The aim of these exercises is to restore this deficiency of cerebromotor impulses. If the exercises are to be carried out properly, I repeat, the teacher must practise all the exercises at the same time as the pupils, however tiring this may be.

Exercise 1: Start with the simplest of these exercises:

(a) Upper limbs   Beat with both hands in 2-time.

    Lower limbs   Strike the floor with alternate feet, with energy and rhythm.

These dissociated movements must be co-ordinated. See that the feet strike the ground at the same time as the hands strike the thighs.

(b) In time with these movements, recite by heart the following consonants:

a–ay–ee–o(pot)–oo–er–wa

and if possible in the reverse order from *wa* to *a*. Very resonant voice. Repeat this exercise 20 times.

Exercise 2: Upright, starting position; legs apart, arms to the sides:

(a) Bend down as far as possible with the arms stretched above the head.

(b) Touch the toes with the hands, then start again, counting aloud.

1! 2! 2! 1! 3! 4! 4! 3!

and so on up to 10, then up to 20, counting each group of figures forwards and backwards.

Exercise 3: Upright position:

Upper limbs	Practise the "squirrel in the cage" exercise at full speed (hands turning over each other).
Lower limbs	Raise the leg, bend the knee and then strike the ground energetically.

In time with these co-ordinated movements, articulate aloud each syllable with slow rhythm: I turn my hands round, I bend my knee (15 times).

Exercise 4: Upright, starting position; legs wide apart, arms extended horizontally:

(a) Place the left hand on the right foot, raising the other arm.

(b) Place the right hand on the left foot, at the same time raising the left arm. Then carry out the exercise in conjunction with the following words, each object to be named aloud, the first syllable to coincide with the movement:

(a) the names of four toys,

(b) the names of four articles used in class,

(c) the four arithmetical operations,

(d) four even pairs of numbers, proceeding from the first to the fourth, then from fourth to first,

(e) four uneven pairs of numbers, treated in the same way,

(f) four geographical terms,

EXAMPLE: mountain, ocean, river, stream.

(g) four names connected with history.

Always proceed from the first to the fourth, then from fourth to first.

Exercise 5: Upright, standing position:

(a) Upper limbs   Hands held sideways at head height (i.e. arm bent at elbow).

Lower limbs   Feet together.

Move the right hand (or left hand in the case of left-handed subjects) forward.

Return the hand to head level, at the same time moving the other hand forward. The two hands should never carry out the same movement. The movement of the one hand forward and the other back should be exactly simultaneous.

(b) Lower limbs   One leg is raised forward and as soon as it is brought back the other is raised.

The same exact simultaneity should be observed for the movement of the legs. As one leg touches the ground the other is raised forward in its place and the exercise is in complete synchronization with the movements of the arms — leg stretched and replaced on the ground, with the arm out — stretched stiffly at the same time.

(c) In time with this exercise, articulate, having memorized the given series of syllables from the first to the last and the last to the first:

ba–bay–bee–bo–boo–bwa–ber, for all the consonants:
k d f g j sh l m n p r s t v x(ks) y z.

Exercise 6: Upright, starting position; legs astride.
(a) Hands joined as if in supplication.

(1) Place the joined hands on the right foot.
(2) Place the joined hands on the left foot.
(3) Raise both arms very high (hands still joined).
(4) Stretch the arms horizontally with hands outstretched.
(5) Bring them back in a forward direction well stretched out, joining the hands together again.

(b) In time with these movements, closely synchronizing the first syllable with the movement, articulate, having memorized the names of the five continents: *Europe, Asia, Africa, America, Australia*. Give a nation or town belonging to each.

EXAMPLE:

Europe	London
Asia	China
Africa	Capetown
America	Washington
Australia	Canberra

A possible alternative is to articulate the names of the five main functions of the body with their principal organ:

Respiration	Lung
Digestion	Stomach
Circulation	Heart
Secretion	Glands
Speech	Larynx

If the teacher possesses a fertile imagination it is legitimate to ring the changes on the words used in this exercise.

Exercise 7: Upright position:

Upper limbs   One hand: bars of 4-time, beaten out with energy and rhythm.

Other hand: military salute, then stretch the arm sideways and strike the thigh (twice).

These dissociated movements must be closely synchronized.

Lower limbs   Energetic steps with alternate feet.

All these movements are to be carried out with vigorous spontaneity.

At the same time as these rhythmic and synchronized movements, we may prescribe (if suitable to the age and cerebral potential of the child):

Repeat digit by digit, forwards and backwards, four-digit numbers, then add up the figures; or spell out in the same way words of four or eight letters.

EXAMPLES: *hand, foot, hour, page, home, time, then*; *palpable, homeless, instinct, importer, armchair*. Practise 20 times.

Exercise 8: Upright, starting position:
Hands at head height, palms toward the teacher (Buddha position).

(a) Clap the hands together.
(b) Stretch the arms sideways.
(c) Raise the arms above the head with the hands outstretched parallel to the sides.
(d) Return the hands to head height, thumbs outwards.

These movements are separated by two beats on the floor with each foot alternately. Two beats with the right, two beats with the left (with energy).

Articulate in time with these movements, having already memorized them, eight names of Asiatic towns or other nouns chosen by the teacher.

EXAMPLES: *Delhi, Peking, Canton, Bangkok, Calcutta, Madras, Hong Kong, Singapore.*

These towns should be articulated from the first to the eighth and from the eighth to the first, then spelt forwards and backwards. Words of academic instructional value should be chosen for this mnemonic exercise.

Exercise 9: Upright position.
Practise the nine movements given below. After five or six periods, the child should have the sequence by heart.

(1) Raise the arms above the head.
(2) Raise and bend the left leg.
(3) Then strike the ground once energetically with that foot.
(4) Extend the right arm horizontally.

9 Speech Disorders

(5) Raise and bend the right leg.

(6) then strike the ground once energetically with that foot.

(7) Raise the left arm above the head (the right arm remaining in the horizontal position).

(8) Clap the hands together above the head.

(9) Lower both arms.

Nine names of the parts of speech should be articulated in exact synchronization, with these movements: *noun, article, adjective, pronoun, verb, adverb, preposition, conjunction, interjection,* as always from the first to the ninth and the ninth to the first. Then spell these words forwards and backwards (without movements).

Exercise 10: Upright position:

Upper limbs   With the flat of the hand strike: one blow on the right thigh, three blows on the left thigh, followed by two blows on the right thigh.

Lower limbs   Movements to conform with those of the hands: one pace to the right, three to the left, one to the right.

In time with these movements, articulate, syllable by syllable the six-syllable words:

Re	in	ves	tig	a	tion
el	ec	tro	the	ra	py
In	sen	si	tiv	it	y

Each of these words should be subsequently spelled forwards and backwards in the normal manner.

Exercise 11: Upright position:

Upper limbs   Right hand: a beat in 4-time

Left hand: a beat in 2-time, i.e. 2 bars of two for each bar of four with the right hand.

Right hand		Left hand	
1	2	1	2
Strike the thigh	Cross the hand on the chest	Strike the thigh	Strike the shoulder
3	4		
Stretch the arm sideways	Strike the shoulder		

Lower limbs: Alternate taps with left and right foot.

Co-ordination of dissociated movements is not easy to start with, but perseverance is essential, since the end can always be achieved, if the exercise is properly conducted.

In time with these movements the pupil should articulate words of two and four syllables, chosen to conform with the beat of the hands:

bar	gain,	ba	ro	met	er
nec	tar,	nu	mis	mat	ic
pen	cil,	de	tcr	min	ant
win	dow,	a	ro	mat	ic
etc.					

Exercise 12: Upright position:

Upper limbs   1. Hands joined, fingers interlaced.

                     2. Stretch the arms sideways.

                     3. Strike the thighs.

Lower limbs   1. Raise one leg forwards.

                     2. Bend the knee.

                     3. Strike the floor with alternate feet.

The movements are then co-ordinated and subsequently practised *with the eyes shut*.

Articulate such phrases as:

"I must speak slowly and clearly articulating every syllable" or enumerate the months of the year from January to December and in the reverse order.

As can be seen, it is easy to create a wide variety of exercises on this basis.

Exercise 13: Upright position:

In addition to developing the rhythm and power of the vocal delivery this exercise is designed to amuse the child. The "exercise game" is based on the imitation of the rolling of a drum. The child is made to imagine himself a member of the regimental bugle and drum band, which is marching past the regimental colours. The band is heard far off, approaching gradually, until it is quite close, then withdrawing gradually into the distance. The pupil holds imaginary drumsticks in his hands and beats out a regular rhythm on the taut skin of the drum.

At the same time he imitates phonetically, at first in a whisper, then progressively louder, the normal rhythmic cadence of a drumbeat. The syllables are clearly separated and very vibrant.

$$rran! \quad rrran! \quad rrran! \quad tan! \quad tan!$$
$$(1) \quad\quad (2) \quad\quad (1) \quad\quad (2) \quad\quad (3)$$

This has the further great advantage of familiarizing the child with the binary (2-beat) and ternary (3-beat) rhythms.

The teacher should himself take part in the exercises as well as controlling it.

The child attacks the sound very quietly at first, with the drumbeat barely audible, then, with increasing vocal power, as the band begins to approach closer and closer to the colours. The voice must ring out clear as the band passes the regimental colours.

The vibrant *r* must be full of enthusiasm! The face shines with radiant happiness, then the sound gradually diminishes. The band moves further and further from the colours and the voice slowly dies away to a whisper.

Practise this exercise 10 times. It is usually a great favourite with the pupil.

Exercise 14: Upright position; feet together:

(a) Extend the right arm horizontally, at the same time crossing the left foot over the right.

(b) Extend the left arm horizontally, returning the left foot to its original position.

(c) Lower both arms, crossing the right foot over the left.

(d) Clap the hands, returning the right foot to its original position.

(e) In strict synchronization with these movements, articulate the various dance terms:

ballet, gavotte, minuet, pavane, waltz, polka, two-step, fox-trot.

The pupil must learn to carry out this exercise with grace, elegance and rhythm. When crossing one foot over the other, the toe must be pointed. The words must be learnt by heart, forwards and backwards, then spelt, forwards and backwards.

Practise 10 times.

Exercise 15: Upright position:

Starting position: arms stretched out in front.

(a) Upper limbs
1. Clench the fists.
2. Open the hands.
3. Spread out the fingers of the right hand, leaving the thumb and index finger close together and bring the hand over to the left hand.
4. As for 3 with the left hand.
5. Spread out the fingers of both hands.

Lower limbs   Strike three forceful steps with the right foot.
Strike three forceful steps with the left foot.

A co-ordination exercise difficult to master initially.

(b) Strictly co-ordinated with the above movements, one word per movement, articulate a number of antonyms (words and their opposites in meaning):

EXAMPLES: hot — cold, long — short, light — dark, broad — narrow, sincerity — hyprocrisy, poverty — wealth, silent — noisy, industrious — lazy, good — bad, fresh — stale.

An extremely important point is to ensure that during every session (at home) the pupil practises the exercises designed to render supple the muscles of the face, the organs of respiration and articulation and does this with the care which athletes devote to their training. It is as pointless to suggest to a subject with a speech impediment, a "speech cripple", whatever the nature of the particular defect, that he should articulate correctly, as to tell a hunch-back to stand up straight.

EXERCISES IN THE LYING-DOWN POSITION

The exercises performed in the lying position are aimed principally at achieving control of the respiratory movements.

The person who stammers must learn to develop a type of combined diaphragm and abdominal breathing. This is the "enlarged" respiration, used by all athletes and singers. These exercises can be carried out even if the child is already performing exercises with the Respirator. The principal aim of the exercise described below is to control the level and volume of the expiration.

The teacher should start by checking the accuracy of the child's motor function in inspiration and expiration. Some subjects find it difficult to expand in one movement the lower part of the cage of the thorax and the abdominal cavity, in order to ensure the complete lowering of the diaphragm. They frequently carry out a clumsy movement by "raising the shoulders"; and this must be resisted. It is the "inverted" respiration, so often found in girls. The expiration movement should be slow, rhythmic and profound, controlled by the muscles of the "abdominal belt": large vertical, large oblique, small oblique and transverse muscles, which as they retract, slowly effect the complete elevation of the diaphragm.

The exercises in the lying position also tone up the abdominal muscles. The motor co-ordination work provides in addition salutary physical and psychic training. Some children have never performed gymnastic exercises; sometimes they are opposed to physical exercise. The performance of my exercises will make them more sure of themselves, with greater control over their movements, more resolute, stronger in themselves.

Exercise 1: Lying position (on the back):

Arms by the sides. Body completely relaxed.

The orthophonic teacher orders "Breathe in" and checks that the movement is properly carried out. The breath is then held and the pupil remains in the inspiration position while the teacher counts up to twelve or fifteen according to the pupil's powers of resistance. This is the respiratory "pause". Then he gives the order: "Blow" and the child blows with all his force, as if he wanted to blow out a candle (12 times).

Exercise 2: Lying position, as before:

On the order of the teacher: rapid, deep and silent inspiration followed immediately by the expiration movement, with a progressive retraction of the abdominal cavity. During the process of expiration the pupil should open the mouth wide and produce a sonorous long *a*, while the teacher counts up to 15, 20, 30 or even higher. A well-trained pupil can hold the *a*, without taking breath, for 50, 60 or 80 half-seconds (10 times). Keep a careful check on the resonance and stability of the sound.

Exercise 3: Lying position:

(a) Lift the right leg.

    Lower the right leg.

    Raise the left leg.

    Lower the left leg.

    Raise the right arm alongside the head.

    Lower the right arm.

    Raise the left arm alongside the head.

    Lower the left arm.

(b) Exactly in time with the above movements, the child should be made to say aloud with correct articulation:

> *I raise* the right leg.
> *I lower* the right leg.
> *I raise* the left leg.
> *I lower* the left leg.
> *I raise* the right arm.
> *I raise* the left arm.
> *I lower* the right arm.
> *I lower* the left arm.

The italicized words should mark the rhythm of the movement being executed.

Exercise 4: Lying position:

(a) Raise both legs simultaneously, without bending, making a straight line from the thighs.

(b) At the same time raise both arms above the head.

(c) Cross the legs.

(d) Separate and spread them.

(e) Bring them together.

(f) Raise both arms and stretch them forwards.

(g) Cross the arms.

(h) Separate them.

(i) Bring them together.

(j) Lower the arms and legs simultaneously.

(k) In exact time with these movements count aloud in tens up to 400 and back again from 400 to 10.

Small children who cannot count in tens should be made to enumerate 10 names of flowers, fruits, or toys, which are easy to articulate. The child should be encouraged to use his own imagination.

Exercise 5: Lying position on the back:

Lower limbs: Bicycle rapidly with legs outstretched.

Upper limbs: The hands rotating round each other in the manner of the squirrel in the cage.

In time with these movements, which are carried out at maximum speed, the stuttering exercise (undifferentiated articulation Exercise 11, p. 121) is practised. The voice must be loud. Continue the exercise without taking a breath. This is the reason for its inclusion in the exercises on respiratory training (10 min per day in two sessions).

Exercise 6: Lying position; body stretched out, arms outstretched above the head:

(a) Swing over to touch the toes without bending the knees.
(b) Lie down again, arms again above the head.
(c) Articulate 20 times:

> I touch my toes.
> I lie back.

Exercise 7: Lying position; arms crossed:

(a) Sit up with the arms still crossed.
(b) Cross the legs like a tailor (Buddha position).
(c) Get on to the knees.
(d) Sit down again with the legs crossed.
(e) Lie down again with arms and legs outstretched.
(f) Articulate in time with the movements:

> I sit up.
> I cross my legs.
> I kneel on my knees.
> I sit down.
> I lie down (10 times).

The teacher must of course help the pupil to carry out this exercise which requires considerable effort.

Exercise 8: Initial position: sitting on the ground, arms extended horizontally, legs spread wide:

(a) Place the right hand on the left foot (raising the other arm).
(b) Then the left arm on the right foot (raising the other arm).
(c) In time with these movements, articulate, having memorized, the names of the marks of punctuation:

.	Full stop	"	Open inverted commas
,	Comma	"	Close inverted commas
;	Semi-colon	-	Hyphen
:	Colon	?	Interrogation mark
··	Dieresis	!	Exclamation mark
'	Apostrophe	...	Ellipse
(	Open brackets		
)	Close brackets		

These should be recited in a loud voice and with clear articulation from the first to the fourteenth and from the fourteenth to the first.

Exercise 9: Semi-lying position:
Forearm on the ground (the position is similar to that normally adopted for sunbathing). Legs about nine inches off the ground. The legs should be stretched out straight with the toes pointed, in order to stretch the legs better.
(a) Slowly raise one leg and lower the other (slightly) toward the ground. Continue with a see-saw motion of both legs.
(b) These movements should be performed in time with an energetic count of one–two, two–one by the teacher, but as if on the pupil's own initiative.

This exercise should be continued as long as the pupil can stand up to it. Although the position has a tonic effect on the abdominal muscles, it is difficult to maintain.

Exercise 10: Same position, but with the legs stretched along the floor, the head and shoulders half way between the sitting and lying positions. The arms are stretched out forwards. The subject must not be allowed to sit up completely since this nullifies the effect of the exercise.

The exercise requires a complete state of immobility during which the subject repeats 10 times in succession the following simple phrase:

I must not move at all (spoken loudly with correct articulation).

Exercise 11: Position — "on all fours":
Perform and at the same time describe in a loud voice the following movements:

(a) I raise the right arm.   (To maintain both arms in the raised
(b) I raise the left arm.   position even for a half-second is
(c) I lower both arms.   difficult).
(d) I stretch out the right leg (on the floor).
(e) I bend the right knee.
(f) I stretch out the left leg.

(g) I bend the left knee.

(h) I stretch out both legs.

(i) I straighten my arms (the straightening of the arms results in the whole of the upper part of the body and the knees being raised).

(j) I bend my elbows.

Go through these movements again from the first to the tenth.

Exercise 12: Lying position on the face, arms stretched out forwards along the ground:

(a) Raise both arms and the upper part of the body.

(b) Lower.

(c) Raise both legs from the thighs.

(d) Lower.

These two movements should be repeated alternately with sufficient rhythm to justify the repetition some ten times of the phrase:

see–saw   see–saw   see–saw

(Try to carry out the exercise 10–20 times).

Exercise 13: Position – sitting on the ground with the legs bent and the knees in the air:

(a) Pass the arms round the knees and hug them firmly.

(b) Lie back flat on the ground.

(c) Come back to the sitting position and remain hugging the knees. See-sawing thus for as long as possible repeat the names of various articles of gymnastic apparatus: *parallel bars, trapeze, rope, rings, vaulting horse, beam, clubs, staves, medicine ball,* etc. As always from one to ten and in reverse from ten to one.

Exercise 14: Position – lying on the back:

(a) In exact synchronization raise the right leg and the left arm and lower them slowly, as if overcoming a heavy resistance.

(b) Carry out the same movements, raising simultaneously the left leg and the right arm.

(c) In time with these movements, articulate the following words 20 times, watching the rhythm.

Note that monosyllabic words are used for raising the limbs and polysyllabic words for lowering.

flower	petunia
(raising)	*(lowering)*
day	inevitable
(raising)	*(lowering)*
work	recreation
(raising)	*(lowering)*
ring	jewellery
(raising)	*(lowering)*
pay	reparation
(raising)	*(lowering)*
lamp	electricity
(raising)	*(lowering)*
pert	imperturbable
(raising)	*(lowering)*
wheat	agriculture
(raising)	*(lowering)*
time	intemperate
(raising)	*(lowering)*
train	locomotive
(raising)	*(lowering)*
show	demonstration
(raising)	*(lowering)*
book	composition
(raising)	*(lowering)*

Practise the movements for all the words. Where twelve words are used, recite them by heart from the first to the twelfth and twelfth to the first.

It is a good thing to have a short conversation with the pupil during each work period. This gives the teacher an opportunity to observe his speech, language and elocution. He should be made to recount little incidents from his daily life, his amusements and his pleasures, say what games he plays (if any), talk about his walks with his parents or days with the Scouts.

It is important for the teacher to know the child's class marks for the month or the quarter, his placing for composition, his successes or failures at school. If possible, a close link between the remedial teacher and the school teacher is always valuable.

Information on the child's behaviour at school and at home are particularly important for the correct orientation and if necessary the modification of the course of treatment. In short the remedial teacher must make the life of his young pupil his very close concern.

For remedial work, affection, an almost maternal interest and real devotion are irreplaceable aids to the energy and technical competence which every worker must possess.

EXAMPLE OF A SESSION OF MULTISENSORY REMEDIAL EDUCATION FOR A CHILD SUFFERING FROM A STAMMER

Sequence of exercise

1. Practise the exercises recorded in the note-book from the previous period. *Correct any errors that may have occurred.*

2. Check the performance of the basic exercises which must be practised every day at home, together with respiration training with the Spirometer.

3. Two new exercises in the sitting position.
One should always include articulation of syllables.

4. Two general co-ordination exercises in the upright position (new).

5. Two exercises in the "lying position".

6. Conversation with the pupil. (From time to time, monthly for example, a short tape recording should be made). Children love to hear the sound of their own voice. It also gives mother, child and teacher a valuable means of assessing the progress of the treatment.

I have not laid down definite rules regarding the number of times these exercises should be practised since this will vary with the circumstances. One exercise may be only slowly mastered, while another may be grasped at once. The teacher must therefore be the judge of how the lesson period is best divided up. Mother and child should never be allowed to leave without the prescribed exercises having been written down in the notebook.

The remedial teacher often finds himself dealing, at home or in hospital, with a large number of child patients. In such cases the children may be grouped by categories, especially those with psycho-neural motor disorders suffering from stammering or stuttering, arhythmia and simple hypotonia.

They can then be treated in groups, especially those of the same age, but not more than twelve pupils should be taken together. The sequence of such collective treatment should follow the order laid down above.

Collective work with its undertones of emulation often has an excellent effect on the psychic state of the child, and this form of treatment can be followed without any harm to the pupils. From the teacher, however, it demands a dynamic approach, closely maintained attention, constant observation and technical competence. In this case we do without the conversation with the pupil and tape recordings.

The child, suffering from speech and language defects, who acquires from these exercises control of his defective cerebro-motor functions, should find himself endowed with a new automatic rhythm in the function of his organs and muscles, which are now ready to obey him and produce the correct phonetic sounds with suppleness and flexibility.

I have given a large number of important examples of these exercises, which the teacher must be prepared to produce from his own imagination in infinite numbers. After more than thirty years as a remedial teacher, I still find it possible to produce almost every day new exercises, adapted to the subject, to his individual disposition, his progress, to his manifestations of will-power and to his neuro-psychic tendencies. In this book I have provided the basic scaffolding on which those who follow me can erect further exercises of every conceivable type.

In serious cases of tonic stammering no signs of progress may appear for a long time, or, worse still, they may appear almost immediately, in which case there is a danger of subsequent relapse. Relapses almost always do occur and must be expected. New instruments have been invented and their sponsors claim to cure stammering in a limited number of periods. How wonderful if this were true – but I remain sceptical. The underlying causes of stammering are too manifold for treatment of any one of them alone to be effective. I only count as positive successes those cases where the improvement is noted at home, at school and in every sphere of life. These results must, moreover, stand the test of time. Only lasting results are in my view valid results. At least fourteen months of work are necessary to effect any improvement in a serious case of stammering. *Results are always achieved quicker with young children which is why it is of such vital importance that the child with a stammer should be treated as soon as the fault is detected.*

I shall never fail to proclaim the truth of this.

It is not part of my purpose to report the forms of medical treatment which can be applied during the process of remedial education. I merely indicate in passing that they are numerous and effective.

THE PSEUDO-NORMAL SUBJECT

It is always curious to observe how long it takes for the human brain to rid itself of certain misconceptions, prejudices and indeed errors. Years of effort are required for false conceptions, based on blindness and ignorance to be put aside. This is a fault to which those charged with the care of the young are specially prone: doctors, nurses, physiotherapists and teachers in particular. In spite of our open condemnation, our work, our prayers, they continue, they persist in following the pernicious policy of waiting for auditory, phonetic, psycho-motor and personality disorders in children to cure themselves.

Sometimes the families themselves are apprehensive regarding the retarded development of their child ... and ask for advice and consultations. Then follows the application of tests and electro-encephalograms, followed by various forms of treatment. The defects naturally get worse; they grow up with the child. When the family are finally brought "by a contact" to a remedial teacher, it is already too late. The child is a prisoner of the school curriculum and the remedial exercises have to be hurried through and therefore neglected. At all costs they must not be allowed to interfere with school lessons or homework. This cannot fail to affect the results of the remedial work.

There is a (large) category of children, suffering from such a variety of broad defects that they defy classification. These subjects are a source of disturbance, upsets, anxiety and trouble at home and at school. There is no apparent disability, either physical or psychic. Their delivery, even when hurried, is normal and so is the voice. They speak a great deal and with assurance. They seem to have wide and coherent interests. Where knowledge fails, imagination steps in. They inspire affection and can be very misleading. Their attention, however, cannot remain fixed on one subject for more than a few minutes. Bantering, showing off, making fun of everything, teasing everyone, the pseudo-normal subject brings his family to the end of its tether. Endowed with definite powers of observation, they love to torment others, refuse all discipline and disdain all adverse comment. The behaviour of such subjects in class varies greatly. In general their teachers find them pleasant, though they rapidly take cognizance of the purposeless activity to which they are given. If the content of the lesson interests him (which is rare) the typical pseudo-normal subject is capable of taking trouble, for he is no fool; out of the blue he gives the right answer to a question or passes up a correct exercise. In essence a clown, he plumes himself on his success, without being able to follow it up. Then we have depression again and relapse. His marks in class are neatly grouped round 0. At home scolding follows reproach. If we trace the fault back, we nearly always find either some hereditary defect or some pathological accident, which has damaged the cerebral motor mechanisms. It may be a case of malaria or alcoholism among the child's ancestors or of a disturbed psychic history in some branch of the family. More generally it is to the prenatal or immediately neo-natal period that the origin of a meningitic condition can be traced. This provides sufficient explanation of the behaviour of these "pseudonormal" subjects. They justify the use of remedial treatment capable of correcting their instability, slow and non-chalant reactions, erring tendencies and the wide variation in their performance at school. These children in addition often find dif-ficulty in writing, reading and arithmetic and sometimes have a suppressed left-handed tendency. Where the intelligence is normal, it is enough for the normal rhythm of activity to be re-established by the training of the cerebro-motor impulses, the will, the capac-ity for self-mastery and the attention for excellent results to be achieved. It is often worthwhile approaching the parents with a view to a modification of their attitude to the child, where neces-sary, and a change in the home atmosphere. There is sometimes friction between brothers and sisters, where there may be right and wrong on both sides and parental intervention can be of use.

In short we must be very wary of these subjects who lay claim to precocious brilliance. It is only a facade and when we penetrate behind the scenes and examine the psychic state of the child, we find cracks, faults and damage, which require urgent repair. These "pseudo-normal" cases are a danger to themselves, to their family, to their future. How many "failures", how many people with grievances and how many good-for-nothings are around, a burden on society! These are the "pseudo-normal" cases who have not been treated while there was still time.

After talking to the child and listening to the complaints of the parents, the child's auditory, phonetic and psycho-neural motor disorders should be traced and recorded (instability, lack of co-ordination, lack of rhythm, academic backwardness, difficulties with reading, writing and arithmetic, a tendency toward perversity of mind and character). These defects are found with particular frequency at the basis of these latter symptoms. Having traced the trouble, the family should be encouraged to show the maximum dignity and firmness toward the child and to avoid the impulse to punish.

The child is then subjected to the various techniques of treatment appropriate to each of these disorders. It is a real duty to bring about contact with the worker in multisensory remedial education, who can to some extent abate the mistakes, misdeeds and failures of these unfortunate creatures, who seem destined for disappointment, despair and perhaps depravity.

PART TWO

Sessions in Remedial Education Designed for the Adolescent and the Adult

CHAPTER VIII

DYSPHONIAS

INFANTILE VOICE —
EUNUCHOID DISABILITY

The retention by adolescents and adults, even after the voice has "broken", of a voice in the treble register is an unhappy and on occasions ludicrous condition. The characteristic feature of this dysphonia is the abnormal pitch of the vocal sounds emitted, which remain well in the treble register.

What is the "breaking" of the voice? It is the change which takes place in the human voice at the period of transition from childhood to adolescence. The period during which the voice breaks is critical; it corresponds to the complete transformation which takes place in the genital organs and the sudden sharp growth of the larynx. It begins to manifest itself toward the age of fourteen in boys and from twelve or thirteen onwards in girls, almost simultaneously with the appearance of the symptoms of puberty, though generally slightly later.

The growth of the larynx occurs very rapidly, especially the diameter from front to rear. The length of the vocal cords increases from fifteen to twenty millimetres in girls and from fifteen to twenty-five millimetres in boys. This results in a complete change of range in the boy's voice; the treble becomes a tenor, baritone or bass and his range falls an octave lower than it was before the breaking of the voice. In the case of the girl the alteration in the voice is considerably less noticeable and the timbre remains very much the same; the voice only drops a couple of tones.

This period lasts for some six months. The voice tends to be raucous, unstable, unpleasant in tone and particularly fragile; abrupt changes in tonal quality give rise to "squeaks" and "cracks". If these defects persist and the physiological modification of the voice is not completed within the normal period of time, remedial exercises should be started in order to effect the lowering of the vocal tone and produce a clear vocal quality.

The muscular system is also affected by this disability of the larynx; the co-operation between the vocal (thyro-arytenoid) muscle loses flexibility resulting in a lack of co-ordination in the tensing and contracting of the lower vocal cords. It is vital to prevent the adolescent misusing and straining his vocal apparatus during the breaking period. The greatest danger of the voice being strained occurs when a group of young boys assemble, burning with enthusiasm for some sporting occasion.

It is obvious that during this critical period the child should be excused any obligation to sing or take part in singing exercises at school. At play and in the family circle he or she should be prevented from any excessive vocal manifestation. A voice which is misused during this physiological crisis becomes hoarse, loses resonance and tonal quality.

When the normal period of time has passed, and a further six to twelve or fifteen months have gone by without any sign of a modification of the voice by a drop in range and by stabilization, the necessary preparations must be made for remedial treatment.

There is usually some psychopathic factor at the root of vocal disorders in the adolescent male. (Such accidents are rare amongst girls). An excessively emotional outlook, fear, "nerves", inhibition, the fear of ridicule are like fetters binding the subject. He no longer dares open his mouth, his breathing becomes periodically spasmodic, the character begins to be affected. The adolescent falls victim to depression, his studies suffer — hence the vital need for action. Such adolescents are frequently sent to me for some very ordinary functional dysphonia, such as hoarseness. One only need listen carefully to the voice to establish the existence of a eunuchoid tendency.

In this case the (remedial treatment) described below, should be applied:

Exercise 1: The subject is seated.

Bring a steady pressure to bear on the thyroid cartilage, so that it slowly but surely drops. Make the subject articulate a long *aaaah* (resonance deep down in the chest). During articulation the larynx should of course be maintained in the lowered position. The boy repeats the long *aaaah* (8 times).

Exercise 2: Make the subject pronounce a short *u* (as in *hut*) then immediately after lowering the larynx: *aaaah*, to make apparent to the pupil the considerable difference between these two phonetic sounds (6 times).

Exercise 3: Keeping the larynx in the lowered position, the subject produces a sustained *aaaah*, while the teacher counts slowly up to 10, 15 or more. This phonetic and respiratory exercise should be repeated six times.

Exercise 4: The subject may now attempt to produce other vowel sounds, without however maintaining the position of the larynx with the hand. The open vowels are practised first: *a–ah–o–or–er–wa* (practise 10 times with close attention to the correctness of the vowel sounds).

Exercise 5: The phonetic vowel sounds are followed by syllables. Begin with the gutturals in conjunction with the vowels:

krarn (with considerable vibration of the *r*)
krang grewa groo grrarn
krree grree (10 times)

Exercise 6: Treat all the consonants in the same way (in the following order):

b p s j sh x(ks) f r l m n z

Each consonant should be practised three times, in conjunction with the vowels given in Exercise 5.

Exercise 7: Practise the following words and expressions: "Good-morning Mrs. Brown. My voice has broken. I can speak in the deeper range".

Vary with quite different words, but in the first place with nasal consonants.

EXAMPLE: equitation

Find large numbers of words ending in *tion, on, ain, er, or*: relation, elocution, notion, repletion, baron, carton, Canton, nylon, train, pain, stain, carter, controller, imitator.

Rembrandt, Rubens, Ramsay, Cardinal Manning, Carron.

Exercise 8: Suggest to the pupil that he should himself produce phrases on the basis of the words which have been practised. They should of course be articulated in the low register.

The pupil should practise twice daily at home for a period of several weeks the vowel *aaaah* and the syllable *arn* in the low register. At least 30 times each syllable. The family must exercise careful supervision over the voice of the young pupil.

The results of the treatment are seen rapidly in most cases. Two or three periods of work are sufficient to effect a transformation of the voice. As in all cases of phonetic therapy, attention must also be paid to the auditory aspect. The ear of the youth with a eunuchoid disorder must become accustomed to the radical change in his voice. This sometimes brings a psychic or nervous reaction in its train. The pupil is disturbed at hearing himself produce a voice which appears to him strange and unaccustomed. I have been able to produce a deeper voice in a matter of minutes (the results of this treatment are sometimes spectacular), but this immediate result has resulted in a flood of tears from the pupil or his mother.

Once the eunuchoid disability has been cured, the defects of character disappear also. The adolescent takes his first steps in the adult world, re-enters the normal school curriculum, he is cured.

It goes without saying that, should the first interview reveal, in addition to these voice defects, one or more dyslalias, they should receive the appropriate type of remedial treatment as soon as the voice has acquired its proper timbre.

A eunuchoid disability, like all other speech defects, never improves with time. Only recently a doctor sent me a patient of forty-nine, suffering from this disability. In a matter of minutes a deeper voice completely new to him had been released. He was amazed and excited.

This is the sequence of remedial treatment.

1. Restore a normal voice to the eunuchoid sufferer.

2. Apply remedial treatment for all other faults including psycho-neural motor defects.

I can only repeat, an isolated disability is rare. It is only too often complicated by other defects.

This must always be remembered if the multisensory treatment is to be effective.

HOARSENESS (LACK OF VOICE)

In tackling the various forms of hoarseness in the adult (aphonias, huskiness), we come up against a complex pathological question. The symptoms vary widely, while there are numerous underlying causes, many of them unsuspected. Hoarseness can be the cause of painful psychopathic conditions and anxiety states. This is justification in itself for our wish to have phonation regarded as the fifth main function of the human body.

Only one who lives, as I have done, in close contact with patients who have lost the power of speech or whose power of self-expression is limited can understand the vital part that speech plays in life.

I have treated patients with aphonias and huskiness of the voice from all social classes, professional speakers and singers, lawyers, doctors, comedians, engineers, teachers, foremen, industrialists, businessmen, churchmen, workmen, nurses, housewives, housekeepers, domestic servants, chauffeurs, taxi-drivers, soldiers, personnel of great organizations, of the railways, of banks, of post offices, etc. All of them, when they fall victim to aphonias and huskiness of the voice, become depressed, worried, cyclothymic, difficult to convince, to encourage, to look after. To apply remedial treatment to these people with functional defects we need a scientific, skilful and psychological approach, we need patience and imagination and above all we must evince an inspiring desire to reassure our patients, to improve their condition, or rather to cure them completely.

I make no mention of methods of treatment for various types of hoarseness, which make use of apparatus, of procedures for deadening the roughness, of electrical massage etc. These are the concern of the medical specialist. Months are required, sometimes a whole year or more, before any positive result is noted, and only then provided that the patient follows exactly the exercises prescribed. No improvement can be held to be valid unless it is confirmed by the oto-laryngolist who has checked that full decongestion of the larynx has been effected and the vocal cords are operating properly.

The causes of aphonias and huskiness of the voice are many and various. The most common are misuse or overstrain of the organs of phonation by public speakers or singers, who make demands on their vocal apparatus in excess of their natural capacity. Schoolmasters and teachers: straining the voice in the course of professional duties. Cause: excessive number of pupils. Ill-directed vocal efforts (in an attempt to be heard above the noise made by 40 to 50 children in a class).

These purely functional speech defects caused by overstrain, result in vocal nodules or in faulty linking of the vocal cords over part or the whole of their length. The vocal cords are no longer in their proper setting *or* the ventricular bands (false vocal cords) are functioning at the expense of the thyroarytenoid muscles (true vocal cords) *or* some mechanical obstacle is obstructing the action of the voice, vocal polypus, cyst on a Morgnani ventricle or some other pathological infection. The treatment in such case is purely medical or surgical.

In this connection it seems useful to provide some statistics for the years 1959–60 and 1960–61.

I gave remedial treatment during this period to twenty-nine patients suffering from functional hoarseness, at the two hospitals where I held consultations: the St. Antoine Hospital (Professor Jacques Debain) and the Lariboisière Hospital (Professor Maurice Aubry).

I had eleven women under observation, divided into the following pathological classes:

One nurse; case of overstrain of the voice in the course of her profession (age 18).

One launderess; case of hoarseness of some years standing; slight inflammation of the vocal cords apparent with glottal cavity (age 33).

One dramatic student, also employed as a telephonist; overstrain (poor setting of the vocal cords) owing to false assumption of a deep voice, speech impediment and inadequate articulation (age 18).

One kindergarten teacher; vocal cords damaged by overstrain in the course of professional duties (age 31).

One secretary; overstrain and misuse of vocal organs; huskiness over a period of 4 years. One nodule: voice strained by group singing (age 30).

Two female mechanics (sisters); vocal strain due to excessive smoking and unruly home background (shouting) (ages 19 and 25).

Two nuns of different orders; vocal overstrain as a result of forcing the voice in ecclesiastical chants (ages 28 and 35).

One shorthand-typist; small larynx, short and narrow vocal cords; speaks with deep tonal quality of the voice with direct contact between the ventricular bands (age 19).

One non-professional woman; psychopathic problems, probably in relation to the menopause (age 45).

Of these eleven I was able to obtain positive improvements in nine cases. Programme of work: one weekly session and three daily practices at home.

Observations on six men:

One lorry driver; recurrent paralysis, misuse and overstrain of the singing voice (age 37).

One railway employee (foreman); functional dysphonia, sudden recurrent aphonias; normal larynx (age 50).

One employee of a commercial firm; paralysis of the larynx as a result of poliomyelitis (age 25).

One workman, a hospital employee; functional dysphonia, dating back to the breaking of the voice. The subject himself admitted that he had "clowned about" with his voice, while singing (age 34).

One adolescent; dysphonia, dating back to premature breaking of the voice (at $12\frac{1}{2}$ years); very nervous type (age 16 years).

One popular singer, who had enjoyed great success; sub-total hoarseness dating back a year. Originally occurred as a result of professional overstrain and a violent fit of anger. Examination of the larynx showed that the subject was speaking with his ventricular bands. The true vocal cords appeared somewhat flabby (age 71).

Results: five cases of definite improvement, one of a year's standing and one showing a very substantial improvement.

Of twelve remaining cases, seven are under treatment, while five have been abandoned.

Occasionally persons have been brought to me suffering from hoarseness of no known functional origin: good setting of the vocal cords, normal larynx and normal respiration. Nothing to note either in the sub-glottal, glottal or super-glottal zones. These are cases of hoarseness of psychic or hormonal origin which are principally found in women.

They have often been sent to me by psychiatrists and oto-laryngologists. Such cases of huskiness require very skilful psychotherapy, based on the exercises given later on. In general, favourable results have been achieved. The results achieved by the remedial treatment depend on:

1. The seriousness of the pathological causes underlying the defects noted.
2. The energy and sagacity of the teacher.
3. The perseverance and discipline of the patient and his attitude of obedience to the exercises prescribed.

I do no more than mention the study of serious pathological causes (diseases of the medulla, paralysis of various origins, cerebral defects, cancer, senility ...). These are the concern only of the medical profession.

One must be a little wary of the enthusiasm manifested by the hoarse patient at the start of the treatment. To escape from the fetters binding his power of expression, he is ready – or believes he is – to make sacrifices. The various forms of therapy applied, including heat treatment, are not making progress and he agrees to undertake these unusual and new exercises. After the treatment has lasted several months the driving energy of the early days begins to evaporate. Courage wavers. It is at this juncture that the teacher must really inject energy into his pupil at every session, restoring his courage, hope and patience in order to obtain his co-operation and active perseverance. This is the critical period, when apathy and indifference threaten the progress of the treatment. It may be necessary to take account of the influence for good or ill of the members of the family circle – a particular husband may either raise or lower his wife's morale, while on the other hand the wife may bring her psychic influence to bear for better or for ill. Parents, children, friends make comments on the results, exaggerating or deprecating the success achieved. All these factors can exercise a favourable or pernicious influence, which the remedial teacher has the thankless task of trying to counter.

Remedial treatment is there to assist the prescribed medical therapy. Regular supervision by a qualified medical specialist is essential in order to check the state of the patient's larynx during the course of the treatment. Collaboration between the medical specialist and the remedial teacher must be continuous. The teacher checks the efficacy of his work as it proceeds. It is the job of the doctor to recommend or advise against heat treatment. The teacher must not exceed his function, he must always operate under the auspices of the oto-laryngologist.

The treatment prescribed for aphonias and hoarseness includes the "basic" exercises, which the patient must practise daily at home, at the beginning of each remedial session. The fresh exercises, prescribed each week by the teacher, are "tailored" to fit the psychic and nervous condition of the pupil. Such a patient may arrive at a remedial session in a state of anxiety, suffering from aphonia, and after a few minutes spent on exercises, may show a definite improvement. The fact is that one must be ready for anything as a remedial teacher and retain one's sang-froid in the face of overflowing enthusiasm or crushing depression. It also needs to be added that even the efforts of doctor and remedial teacher are by no means always crowned with success. There are recalcitrant cases, which is why one must always be very circumspect with the patient and refrain from making promises about the possibility of cure. Fate can make a mockery of the most favourable prognoses.

EXERCISES

Apart from the prescribed exercises, complete vocal abstinence (for both singing and speaking voice) should be imposed on the patient.

1. Respiratory training: aimed at developing and regularizing the inspiration and expiration. Ten minutes respiration (nose and mouth) per day with the "Respirator".

2. Twenty times morning and evening: exercise for "enlarged" respiration in the lying position.

Breathe in silently, dilating the nostrils (rapid movement) without raising the shoulders.

Breathe out very slowly, counting up to 30–35, or more if possible.

These exercises should be carried out daily at home.

3. Training of the organs of articulation. It is of vital importance that the dysphonic patient should articulate the phonetic sounds with energy and precision. This entails the training of the muscles and organs involved in articulation. If any form of dysarthria is present, this should be treated with the appropriate exercises.

(a) Lower the maxilla in one movement, opening wide the lips to the corners.

(b) Close the mouth sharply, bringing the teeth together energetically (30 times morning and evening) (one half-second per movement).

4. Move the maxilla in a sideways direction, opening the mouth (one half-second per movement).

5. (a) Move the maxilla forwards.

(b) Pull the maxilla back sharply, while opening the mouth (one half-second per movement). The mouth should remain open throughout this exercise (20 times morning and evening).

6. (a) In one movement stretch the naso-labial groove (upper lip), opening the mouth at the same time.

(b) Close the mouth sharply, raising the facial muscles towards the eyes (30 times morning and evening).

7. (a) Push the lips forward in exaggerated fashion, as if to articulate *oo*.

(b) Spread wide the lips and cheeks as if in a hearty laugh.

This exercise to be practised silently 30 times morning and evening (one half-second per movement).

8. (a) Open the mouth wide.

(b) Put out the tongue abruptly.

(c) Shut the mouth and clench the teeth.

Practise 20 times morning and evening.

These are the "basic" exercises which the patient must learn once and for all to carry out at home without the teacher having to supervise their practice.

It is of course a good thing to check from time to time that they are being carried out correctly. It does not take long to check correct execution and a practical check is necessary. The teacher, bearing in mind the information provided by the medical specialist on the state of the larynx and the texture of the vocal cords, will to the best of his ability assess the natural voice range of the subject. It is a question of observation, adjustment and careful investigation.

9. Pronounce very lightly and very briefly the vowel *ay* (as in d*a*y) with a sharp tone. Unmusical subjects, who are frequently met with, find it difficult to discriminate between a short, medium

and long stress on a vowel. This difference must be brought home to them by means of examples or by playing F sharp of octave 4 on the piano. Even so they find difficulty in appreciating tonal quality. This is where the teacher's knowledge of physiology and acoustics are of such vital importance. A highly developed auditory sense is required to appreciate even to a "comma"* whether a sound is in tune.

It is worth noting that the victim of hoarseness cannot as a general rule produce an audible note. It is important to explain to him that this is of no significance and that these repeated attempts on the vowel *ay* are only designed to train the vocal cords to link together properly. This vowel, should be sounded sharply like a flick of the fingers, even if it doesn't produce any perceptible sound. Practise the exercise 10 times in succession — after a rest period, varying from a few minutes to half an hour. Repeat ten times during the day.

EXAMPLE: *ay! ay! ay! ay! ay! ay!* Stop and attempt the vowel afresh each time. Open the mouth and separate the lips widely. Repeat 20 times per day the phrase, "I must speak in a very clear voice?" with an interrogative note in the voice.

10. Method as for the previous exercise, brief, short attempts, repeated 10 times during the day, in this case on the vowel *ee*, again in the high range:

ee! ee! ee! ee! ee! ee! (F sharp) mouth open

Corners of the lips parted. Practise 10 times with rest periods in between.

11. Close the mouth tightly (so that the mucous surfaces of the lips are invisible).

Attempt sounds in the high register with the mouth closed, indicating to the patient that during this exercise he should feel sensations of internal vibration behind the incisor block and throughout the face (200 times daily with mouth closed).

---

* The comma is the barely appreciable interval between two notes such as F sharp and G flat.

12. Lightly touch on the vowels *ay! ee!* in succession one after the other in continuous series of 10 (in the high register) *ay! ee! ay! ee! ay! ee! ay! ee!* etc. Practise six times daily.

13. Touch lightly in the high register the vowels *o* (as in h*o*t), *an* (as in c*an*'t) 10 times in succession. Practise six times daily *o! an! o! an! o! an! o! an!* etc.

14. Pronounce in the middle register of the voice in a whispered tone, with a delivery slightly faster than usual, the vowel sounds *aa–ee–ay–o–an*, slurring the sounds into each other. Repeat this slurred series *a–ee–ay–o–an* 10 times. Practise the whole exercise six times per day.

15. Practise the preceding exercise in the "deep" register, but touching each vowel lightly instead of slurring the sounds:

a! ay! ee! o! an! Pay particular attention to the vocal timbre which must be exactly right. Repeat 15 times. Check the tonal quality, which should be uniform for all vowels. It must not deteriorate into an imitation of a fire brigade siren. The interval between the sounds must not be drawn out. This is difficult to bring home to the subject, but it is important. We have to persevere, thinking of melodic rhythm and the intonations which will have to be observed in the spoken voice, when it has become clearer and more expressive.

16. When, and only when, some improvement is noted in the condition of the patient, practise consonants and vowels together.

Initially the vowels should be touched lightly in the high register, in conjunction with the consonants shown:

bay!	*bee!*	*nay!*	*nee!*
kay!	*kee!*	*pay!*	*pee!*
day!	*dee!*	*ray!*	*ree!*
fay!	*fee!*	*say!*	*see!*
quay!	*quee!*	*tay!*	*tee!*
jay!	*jee!*	*vay!*	*vee!*
shay!	*shee!*	*xay!*	*xee!*
lay!	*lee!*	*yay!*	*yee!*
may!	*mee!*	*zay!*	*zee!*

In addition to the correct pitch of the sounds the teacher must of course assess the correctness of the articulation of all the consonants, although this will naturally have been done at the start of the treatment of the dysphonic patient.

17. Practise very briefly and lightly clearing the throat deep down, opening the mouth wide and separating the corners of the lips (60 times daily in three sessions).

18. Touch lightly in low, middle and high registers, all the vowel sounds in succession.

EXAMPLE:　　　　　　　*a!*　　*a!*　　*a!*
　　　　　　　　　　　 low　middle　high

and still on the same vowel, come down from the high to the low register:

　　　　　　　　　　　　a!　　*a!*　　*a!*
　　　　　　　　　　　　high　middle　low

The terms "high", "middle" and "low" are of course adapted:

(a) to the male or female voice (the male voice is an octave lower than the female voice);

(b) to the voice-range of the individual;

(c) to the degree of improvement, already achieved in the condition of the patient's voice. These exercises should be practised progressively in the light of the rate of recovery of the patient.

This exercise includes all the other vowels, which have to be practised in the same way as: *a! ay! ee! o!* (as in p*o*t) *oo! wa! er! wee!*

It is not possible to practise all these vowels in the course of a single session; they should be worked over four at a time in the three registers. One should always beware of tiring the patient.

19. If the condition of the patient's larynx allows and if he is articulating the sounds correctly and precisely, an attempt may be made to increase the power of his voice, but this phase of the treatment must be handled very delicately. Constant checks must be carried out during the process of the psycho-motor education of these dysphonic patients. Prudence is essential; a too rapid ad-

vance can be dangerous and might lead to a relapse. This should be avoided.

It should never be forgotten that the co-ordination of the vocal cords is controlled by the cerebro-motor mechanisms and in particular by the recurrent nerve. The neuro-psychic state of the patient must therefore be kept under supervision.

In order to develop the intensity of the voice, the patient is made to articulate, at first in a whisper and then in a more resonant tone, the syllables:

ga! gan! goua!

articulated with energy and attack. The vocal intensity is gradually reduced down to a whisper again. Even at the whispered intensity the articulation must lose none of its precision. This must also be carefully checked. Practise these syllables 20 times.

It is an excellent practice to make frequent tape recordings since the pupil likes to hear the sound of his own voice and assess his progress.

20. We still practise the production of the vowels, lightly and in the high register:

ay ee ah

At the beginning of the period the pupil should be made to practise silently the exercise which I have called "stuttering" (frantic movement of the tongue inside the mouth, coupled with similar movement of the lips and cheeks) (5 to 6 minutes per day).

21. Practise a slight clearing of the throat at the base, pronouncing the syllable *rroo*

the syllable *ghee* (hard *g*)

Divide this exercise which is carried out in the normal voice and with normal resonance, into three movements, beaten out by the hands as follows:

1	2	3
Strike the knees	Stretch the arms sideways	Strike the shoulders

Practise 20 times, provided the patient does not become tired.

It is a good thing to attempt to combine speech with mimicry, since mimicry is really a second language which, almost as much as articulation, comes to the aid of the spoken word to complete its meaning.

EXAMPLE: (for the expressive articulation of a very simple phrase).
This little boy is charming and sensible...
It's a pity he does not talk...

First idea: vivacious tone to express the charm and intelligence of the child, followed by: the imitation of the development of sorrow and regret, which prepares the way for the expression of the second idea.
Second idea: it's a pity that he does not talk...

Passing from the gay happy subject of the first idea to the second idea the liveliness of the expression fades, accompanied by a general drooping of the facial muscles. The language of mimicry is invoked to indicate the passage from one idea to the next.

For all human beings, expression by means of mimicry adds a further dimension to the spoken idea; it indicates the direction which an idea is taking and evokes a thought that mere words are powerless to express.

In the case of persons suffering, for whatever reason, from defects of speech or articulation, expression by means of mimicry assumes a more marked importance.

Not all human beings are by nature expressive. The apathetic, the victims of ataraxia, the egocentrics most often lack the power of expressive mimicry. Race and place of origin play a role in this. Southerners are more expressive than people from the North. The expressive gestures and the mimic powers are, for example, far more highly developed among the men of Provence than among the Flemish peoples. The phlegmatic Englishman is a by-word.

It is of advantage to train our dysphonic patients in the art of expression by mimicry which is as capable as its related function, articulation, of taking the place of vocal intensity and economizing as far as possible the effort spent on speech.

22. The pupil is asked to produce very simple words or phrases, centred round an idea of his own choice. This also helps to develop the imagination.

Let us assume that some such phrase as the following has been produced:

We are intending to travel during our holidays.

The pupil learns by heart and articulates correctly and with precision this phrase five or six times. The teacher then asks him to speak the same phrase, endowing it with the intonation appropriate to the following feelings:

Dismay	Pity
Pleasure and delight	Regret and remorse
Doubt and distrust	Ardent hope
Authority that brooks no dispute	Entreaty
Nostalgia	Triumph

and, the most difficult of all to interpret:

Complete indifference.

As can be seen, it is possible to evoke the whole range of human emotions. The difficult point is to impart them to the same phrase, which has no immediate connection with the particular emotion. In this case, however, a maximum demand is made on the cerebral mechanism of the pupil. To evoke, with the aid of a single banal phrase, the shade of meaning and the intonation appropriate to the prescribed sentiment is difficult beyond all dispute. It does, however, constitute a beneficial and intense form of training for the psycho-motor cerebral mechanisms.

23. The hoarse patient, once he has achieved an almost normal degree of automatism in speech and articulation, should be made to practise daily, either alone in front of a mirror or in the presence of members of his family, short conversations (6–7 minutes) on subjects which are always different and require improvisation. In his everyday life the dysphonic patient should be advised to abandon his "vocal abstinence" with caution and with method. He must avoid shouting or straining his vocal apparatus, especial-

ly where people are smoking. For the vocal organs other peoples' smoke is even more harmful than one's own.

24. The hoarse patient should practise speaking for as long as possible during the same expiration. He should be made to articulate long phrases with little breathing, speaking very slowly.

EXAMPLE: *I must articulate clearly, in order to avoid tiring my larynx and straining my voice.*

The delivery of this phrase should not be hurried; it should if necessary be repeated twice during the one expiration (practise 10 times).

In the rare cases (outside the singing profession), where the dysphonic patient who has recovered his vocal resonance displays any possibility of being able to sing again, singing exercises over a very short range should be very cautiously undertaken: three notes: thirds or fourths or chromatic scales over this range; (span of four notes), in fifths: (five notes) as for a piano exercise, up and down, on the vowel *ah*. Exercises should be practised very slowly, over a limited range. Never exceed an octave, i.e. an interval of eight tones.

"Passages" i.e. transitions from lower to medium or medium to upper register must be watched with particular care. If the voice is stable and homogeneous and the pitch correct, the singing training may be continued, but never too fast initially. Prudence, above all, prudence is required.

I have on occasions been surprised to find a voice of good timbre re-emerge. This method of multisensory remedial education has produced excellent results. It is, however, important to avoid singing in an incorrect range! This can lead to very serious consequences. In fact voices of unlimited range simply do not exist. If one takes as a criterion even those laid down by oto-laryngologists, composers and numerous teachers of singing one runs the risk of dangerous errors. The register and timbre of the voice are as individual as the individual himself! It is permissible to work on the range and stability of the singing voice, but not on the natural range, and still less on the timbre of the voice!

The teacher teaches (if he is capable of doing so) and advises but it is the voice which accepts or rejects the teaching. It grows, becomes stronger and more stable, or it fades and loses its keen edge; these are the only criteria that can be used in the science of teaching singing, and I might add in that of teaching speech.

The stages in the remedial treatment of adult cases of hoarseness:

Stage one

1. Respiration exercises with and without respiration apparatus.
2. The "basic" exercises (maxilla, lips, tongue) (preparatory to articulation).
3. Very light, brief attempts on the short *ay* (as in *day*) in the high register.
4. High sounds with the mouth closed.
5. Very light, brief attempts on the vowel *ee* in the high register.
6. Articulate almost in a low voice (with tonal quality similar to that of a little girl or boy) and with an interrogative tone: "I must speak in a very clear voice?" (20 times per day).

The first stage should last at least two weeks, at the end of which an examination by a medical specialist should be insisted on.

Stage two

Initially the same exercises as in Stage one. Then add:

1. Attempts made lightly and in the high register on the vowels *o! an!* as indicated in Exercise 13.
2. Produce lightly, one after the other but detached, the vowels *ay! ee!* (Exercise 12).
3. A few minutes silent "stuttering".
4. Light clearing of the throat at the base.
   The second stage should last 20–25 days.
   The condition of the larynx should be checked by a specialist.

Stage three

All the exercises contained in Stage one.

1. Lightly touch on the vowel *aa* in all three registers and, in fours, the vowels in the other series.

2. Carry out Exercises 13, 14, 15 and 16; never more than four during the one period.

According to the progress of the treatment, this stage should only be begun after two to two and a half months of treatment.

As soon as any improvement in the form of decongestion, coupled with recovered elasticity and tonus of the vocal cords, has been established by the medical specialist, prescribe Exercises 16–22, ringing the changes on them according to the physical and psychic condition of the pupil. At this point an examination by a laryngologist is necessary in order to decide whether the treatment should be intensified or continued with moderation.

I cannot emphasize too strongly that remedial workers of both sexes must be adroit, shrewd and tactful in the practice of very delicate methods for a psychotherapy which is skilful and effective. They must be able to reassure, to encourage and at the same time bring home to their patients the need for perseverance, courage and methodical work.

Many hoarse patients (in addition to professional singers), whom we can introduce to techniques destined to save them, come to us exceedingly disturbed and even in a state of anxiety. These are the teachers from primary schools and indeed all who follow the teaching profession. The average vocal equipment of a teacher, man or woman, cannot hope to compete with the overwhelming numbers of pupils in the classes of primary, secondary and higher educational establishments. I have been deeply moved by some of the things teachers have said to me.

Girls who have devoted their youth and contributed their money (or their parents' money) to preparing themselves for a career to which they feel drawn by a feeling of vocation, by that mixture, peculiarly feminine, of an almost maternal devotion, of knowledge, of skill, of competence and by the constant inner drive toward self-sacrifice.

Justice has not always been done to the body of teachers, whether public or private. This is a glaring error. If there are occasionally bad shepherds, the majority serve the community well, as I have often found.

I have the highest regard for social assistants and mistresses at primary schools. Our professional paths run side by side and we often need to exchange information and views. The fact is that families sometimes fail to appreciate the teacher and do not hold them in the respect and affection to which they are entitled. I have seen at close quarters the despair of young dysphonic patients (teachers at public or private schools) at the idea of having to abandon what they regard as a sacred duty. We need all our love, all our fraternal feeling and devotion to raise them from the slough of despondency.

I have had the good fortune in certain cases to alleviate their bitter sorrow and allow them an opportunity of regaining their school positions or in other cases to take their courses again. If only for this I maintain that multisensory remedial education justifies every sacrifice and that it is in fact one of the finest causes to which a woman can devote herself.

NASAL TWANG AND NEGATIVE NASALITY (DENASALIZATION)

These forms of dysphonia are far less serious than hoarseness. Certain adults, however, have managed to carry over from the speech of their childhood an irritating nasal twang (which has been left untreated or has been treated badly), which is unpleasant to hear and may prove an impediment in their family or professional life.

The nasal twang in the speech of an adult may have originated in a bad habit, contracted in childhood sometimes by mimicry, or be the result of an anatomic lesion or malformation, crack or performation of the palate arch, division of the velum, hare lip, centrally-sited paralysis, paresis of traumatic origin, or of some mechanical obstacle to the normal flow of resonance, such as over-developed adenoids, or obstruction of the cavum.

Such forms of nasal twang are only rarely found in adults. Medical therapy and surgical intervention have to some extent removed the mechanical causes, lesions, malformations etc. in childhood. There remains only the most frequent category, cases where a bad habit has not been eliminated by remedial treatment in infancy or childhood.

Staphylorrhaphy or uranostaphylorrhaphy have very little effect on the speech of the patient. Remedial education is the indispensable complement to the operation in order to exploit to the full the anatomical results achieved. The earlier surgical intervention and orthophonic therapy is applied, the more effective the recovery of speech will be. In fact the nasal twang in adults is rare.

We do find forms of negative nasality (denasalization) which should have received remedial treatment in childhood. Unfortunately the reasons — and the results — are always the same. "It will pass", "it will sort itself out" was heard too often at the age when remedial treatment should have been applied. As a result we are called on to treat adults who, when the dysphonia is pronounced, have nasal voices like the voice of Punch.

These nasal qualities are particularly difficult for singers and comedians. Others may not worry about their disability unless someone of importance draws their attention to it. In such cases a tape recording can be beneficial. As the Abbé Millet, our master in phonetics, remarked, with his characteristically simple approach, "The ear learns from the mouth". This is entirely true as one finds when trying to correct a regional or foreign accent. I may point out that women of what it is customary to call "high society" (why this nomenclature?) frequently affect a nasal quality. They are fewer in number than they used to be, but they preserve an unfortunate manner of speaking and endow their speech with a veneer of snobbery. Here are their faults:

1. Habitual pitching of the voice in the high register irrespective of its natural range.
2. Defective articulation.
3. Too rapid diction.
4. Nasal quality (acquired by mimicry); what is called the "salon voice", with latent dysphonia and often dysarthria. For this, however, there is no cure and down the generations the mimicry of family and caste continues to hold sway.

Remedial treatment is the same for nasal twang and nasal quality. The paramount aim is to foster the tone and mobility of tongue and velum.

The contractions of the wall of the pharynx during speech must be eliminated and the ear must be educated to accept a voice free of its predominant nasal resonance.

EXERCISES

Exercise 1: Nasal and buccal (mouth) respiration training, using the "respirator".

Exercise 2: Lower the maxilla sharply and, keeping it lowered, articulate clearly 40 times the open *a* (as in *hark*) sharply and with resonance, without contracting the pharynx.

Exercise 3: Protrude the lips in exaggerated fashion, shouting: *ah.*
Open them widely, shouting: *arn.*
Practise this exercise forty times.

Exercise 4: With mouth open wide, showing the corners of the lips fully, carry out violent clearing of the back of the throat. 150 times per day.

Exercise 5: Articulate 50 times (precisely and sharply):

ja! shay! torn!

Divide these syllables up by a measure of 3 times, beaten out with energy by the outstretched hands.

Exercise 6: Clear the throat violently, followed immediately, with the mouth still open, by a forceful attack on the syllables:

kron–kree–krer

Exercise 7: As for Exercise 6, but articulating the voiced guttural *g* in place of the unvoiced guttural *k*:

grra! gree! grer!

Exercise 8: If the nasal twang shows signs of diminishing after seven or eight sessions and twice daily practice, practise at home in a loud voice whole series of syllables with consonants and vowels: *ba–bay–ber–bwa–bwee* and for all the consonants: *k–d–f–g–j–sh–l–m–n–p–r–s–t–v–x(ks)–y–z.*

Exercise 9: Practise the two phonetic sounds *se* and *ze*, which are rarely articulated correctly by such dysphonia subjects.

assa! ass! aza! az! (40 times) then the same exercise, substituting the following vowels for the *a*:

eessee	*eess*	Forty times. Pay particular attention to
eezee	*eez*	the correct articulation of the conso-
oosso	*ooz*	nants and the correct timbre of the vow-
ooswee	*weez*	els.

Exercise 10: Articulate the following associations of consonants and vowels, taking care to avoid contraction of the pharynx, the palatal velum and the base of the tongue:

kra–kla–kssa	Articulate each group of syllables ten
bra–bla–bza	times.
gra–gla–gza	
zhla–zhra–zhsa	
shla–shra–shsa	
fla–fra–fsa	
vla–vra–vza	
pla–pra–psa	
sla–sra–zla	
zra–kssra–gazra	
dla–dra–dza	
tla–tra–tsa	

Exercise 11: Articulate the same phonetic sounds in the weak position:

akr–akl–akss	Articulate each group of syllables ten
abr–abl–abz	times.
agr–agl–agz	

azhl–azhr–azhs
ashl–ashr–ashs
afl–afr–afs
azr–arrsk–azzg
avl–avr–avz
apl–apr–aps
asl–asr–azl
asd–ard–azd
ast–art–azt

Exercise 12: Practise Exercises 10 and 11 with the normal series of vowels:

ay–ee–o–oo–wa–er–wee.

Exercise 13: It is useful to practise syllables, in which the nasal twang and negative nasality have to be suppressed in the body of the word. To exercise his imagination, the subject should be made to find the words himself.

EXAMPLES: *arbour, Alaska, exhaust, exhale, inhale, eagle, creature, gaffer, flat, torpedo, Africa, cape, group, slave, Jasper, hardy.*

The pupil should be asked to build phrases around words which he has been given, or which he has himself produced.

Exercise 14: Once a degree of automatism has been acquired in speech, make the pupil give a short talk every day (this must be done at home as well). It should be planned to last a few minutes and be done on the spur of the moment. I prefer this type of work to reading aloud. Since speech, articulation and language are the result of psycho-neural and motor effort, it is desirable to train the cerebromotor mechanisms. Reading is a passive occupation, which does not afford the multisensory training which our techniques of remedial teaching seek to inspire.

Exercises for the correction of nasal twang and nasal qualities should follow the sequence, form, content and number which I have just described.

PHONASTHENIAS

These are functional disorders affecting the synergic muscular activity which plays a part in the production of voice, articulation and language. The vocal power is sensibly diminished. The patient murmurs his words in a completely altered voice which, although not hoarse, is barely audible. It is due to a psychomotor defect localized in the organs of phonation and articulation.

Phonasthenias are normally psychopathic in origin and fall within the province of the oto-laryngologist and the psychiatrist. They are sometimes caused by neuropathic disorders, such as general paralysis, multiple sclerosis, Little's syndrome, Parkinson's disease, cerebellar syndrome or encephalitic disease. In these serious cases the changes in articulation and language lie outside the scope of multisensory remedial education. A hearing defect may result in the introduction of a flat deadened quality of the voice. This also requires examination by a medical specialist.

There are, however, some types of phonasthenia of psychoneural origin, for which we can apply useful corrective treatment. A sudden fright, inhibition, psychic trauma, terror, grief may give rise to a state of motor constraint in the speech organs and produce spasms, extending even to the motor system of the diaphragm and the whole of the respiratory system.

Remedial teachers have little contact with this type of patient who requires medical treatment.

If one is faced with functional disorders of this nature, it is a good thing to try to trace the root cause, to reassure the patient, raise his morale and only refer very occasionally to the disability, from which he is suffering. Tests for deafness will have been applied and we can, therefore, omit them. If this form of vocal inhibition is of psychic origin, the psycho-neural motor exercises may prove decisive. I must repeat, however, that a remedial teacher cannot treat patients of this type unless referred to him by a qualified doctor.

I may add that it is worth remembering that cases of simulated disability have been known.

Exercise 1: The patient lies on his back on the floor in a darkened room (if it is light) with the curtains slightly drawn. A small flat cushion is placed under his head. Make him breathe in deeply, rapidly and silently through the nose (the base of the thorax and the abdominal cavity should be dilated in a single movement). The movement of expiration is then carried out: very slowly, very quietly, very rhythmically, breathing out through the mouth and progressively retracting the abdomen. The teacher kneels beside his pupil.

Practise this silent breathing 6 times.

Exercise 2: Inspiration as before. The expiration movement begins with a simple breath, but with the slow steady whispering of the phrase.

Heavens, how well I breathe!

This phrase to be articulated ten times slowly and with conviction.

Exercise 3: Rapid and silent inspiration. The phrase is changed slightly:

O how calm I feel.

Repeat this 15 times.

My heart beats evenly and steadily.

Speak slowly. Instil into the pupil the feeling of well-being, inherent in these phrases.

Exercise 4: Suggest that the patient shut his eyes. The teacher then counts slowly from "1 to 100" and from "100 to 1".

Contrary to what might be expected, the pupil remains awake, while the teacher is counting from 1 to 100. He is calm, relaxed and at peace.

Exercise 5: The patient at the request of the teacher, recalls some scene and describes it in a low voice.

This exercise is similar to one prescribed for psycho-neural motor disorders: inhibited subjects, tonic stammerers, stutterers, choreic patients.

EXAMPLE: You are in the country in the middle of a garden which has a lawn. Put yourself in the place of someone in the garden and describe what you see and the person you are with or the people around you. Are there any children? What are they like? The teacher must help his pupil and unobtrusively prompt him to recall and relate what he sees to the best of his ability. The imagination of teacher and pupil can create an infinite number of exercises of this type.

Exercise 6: The pupil then repeats a further fifteen times the phrase: "Oh how easily I breathe!" "I am so very calm". The teacher then tells the pupil to close his eyes again and counts (still in a low voice) from 1 to 100 and from 100 to 1.

Exercise 7: The pupil sits up quietly and remains in the sitting position, while the teacher illuminates the room. The pupil then stands upright and carries out the following movements: arms and legs apart, rotate the trunk as far as possible to the right and left. Tempo: One second per movement.

In time with each movement, the pupil repeats eight or ten nouns, taken from the scene described in Exercise 5. These nouns are spoken from the first to the last and then in the reverse order. Practise 10 times.

Exercise 8: Make the pupil clear the throat violently thirty times at the base of the throat, opening the mouth wide, until the corners of the lips show.

Exercise 9: Make the pupil beat out (in the sitting position) bars of 2-time, in time with dissociated movements.

Strike the shoulder with one hand, while the other strikes the knee and vice versa.

Again in time with these exact and forceful movements, make the pupil articulate as loudly as possible:

agrer! agrer! (30 times).

Exercise 10: Practise the non-differentiated articulation exercise (as fast as possible). Frenzied movement of the tongue inside the mouth, coupled with large-scale lip and cheek movement. Attempt to add sound to this exercise for a few minutes, then practise for 10 minutes per day at home.

Exercise 11: The pupil is made to articulate three consecutive words, first in a very low voice, then very loudly. Practise 20 times each way.

EXAMPLES: *violin–piano–bassoon,*
                     hotel–resort–vacation,
                     courage–energy–enthusiasm.

If it is loud enough to be audible, the voice should be recorded on a tape recorder. This provides an excellent method of bringing home to the patient himself his lack of vocal tone and whatever progress is being made. This is at once an encouragement and a stimulus to further effort.

Exercise 12: It is permissible to vary the phrases articulated in a position of relaxation, and also the co-ordination and phonetic exercises. What I have outlined above is the plan of a remedial session. The sequence should be observed. The pupil should be instructed to practise at home the respiration exercises with phrases and then the phonetic exercises in sitting and standing positions. Never omit the undifferentiated articulation exercise.

Appreciable progress can normally be observed after three or four weeks; everything depends on the patient, his energy and his determination to recover a normal voice.

We know of families in which all the members mumble inaudibly. This is a collective habit based on imitation. Deaf people in such families are in an especially unfortunate plight.

CHAPTER IX

DYSARTHRIA IN THE ADULT

IN PRINCIPLE, an adult, suffering from one or more dysarthrias, remains almost unaffected by his disability, if indeed he is aware of it. He should of course have received remedial treatment in infancy. Ignorance or negligence have deprived him of this. If he comes for advice it will be because some member of his circle has made fun of him and pointed out the absurdity of his speech.

It can be observed that dyslalic patients abound in the streets and only a minute proportion receive remedial treatment, that only phonetic troubles which actively impede the exercise of a profession claim any attention, that it is only when "there is no alternative" that people cry "Help".

Adults, does it need to be said, are far more difficult to re-educate than children. With a child, in ninety-nine cases out of a hundred there is a relatively favourable response to discipline; it does not take long for the authority of voice and eye to exact obedience. The adult, however, holds back. Either he makes light of his speech and its defects (and works without conviction) or his self-respect suffers and he becomes cantankerous. In either case we have to fight, struggle, tame and conquer our patient — not always an easy task. The pupil will discuss and comment and lose himself in false theorizing. It needs great skill to bring him into a frame of mind where he will trust and accept the teacher and the teaching. He is, moreover, bound by his professional obligations with their strict time-table. If he agrees to undertake remedial treatment, he is only prepared to devote a very limited time to his exercises at home. For the teacher it is often a thankless task, destined to failure, difficulty and disappointment... but the harder the task, the more praiseworthy our efforts.

Do we not know numbers of dyslalic patients who have remained prisoners to their disability, and with their diplomas, their positions, their honours, still speak in a manner quite grotesque? To hear, for example, a learned lawyer "lisp" is a sore blow for a phonetic specialist. These important persons give lectures, moreover, and their services are in great demand. They may suffer from a vocal disability, which resists victoriously the amplification of the microphone. Their articulation may be inadequate or bad, involving defective sibilants and gutturals which are missing or else over-emphasized. They may possess regional accents, which deprive their language of distinction. The public whom they are addressing hear nothing, as words and meaning are lost in the jumble of sound, the confusing jabber, which they can barely decipher. Nevertheless they applaud "at the end". They applaud the distinguished forehead, which houses a famous brain, the uniform and decorations which deck the person. As to his speech, that is left out of account; speech is the "poor relation".

Is it then completely impossible to bring home to these "stammering", "stuttering" people how sad it is that no one can hear the remarkable pronouncements which they lavish on the world, to persuade them how much better it would be for them to employ a "speaker", who would make known to enthusiastic and interested audiences the fruits of their work and researches. Logic is, alas, seldom appreciated.

THE LISP

The alteration in the articulation of the unvoiced and voiced sibilant consonants s and z is commonly known by the onomatopoeic name of lisping. Its causes are multiple:

(a) A left-handed tendency repressed in early childhood.
(b) A slight hearing defect, which has escaped notice.
(c) Maxillary atresia and defective spacing of the teeth.
(d) Bad habits acquired by mimicry within the family circle.

Whatever the causes may be the remedial treatment for a lisp is the same.

The hearing should be checked by a laryngologist who will arrange for the taking of an audiogram. Investigate the possibility of a left-handed tendency and practise co-ordination exercises, especially with the left hand. The advice of a specialist in mouth formation should be sought regarding the use of corrective equipment and dental aids.

Draw the attention of the adult patient suffering from a lisp, to the infectious nature of the lisp. Very often lisping children have been brought to me by mothers who lisp equally badly.

REMEDIAL TREATMENT

Exercise 1: The subject should be taught the various "basic" exercises, which I have described several times in this book (not forgetting the clearing of the throat and respiration through nose and mouth with the "respirator").

Add the following:

(a) Clench the teeth with the lips wide open.
(b) Open them sharply. Practise 40 times, articulating very loudly:

da ta na

taking care not to introduce the top of the tongue between the incisors.

Divide the above exercise among the following movements:

(1) Strike the breast with hands well spread.
(2) Fling the arms sharply sideways (for left-handed subjects, use the left hand only).
(3) Strike the knees.

Exercise 2:

(a) Clench the teeth.
(b) Whistle *sss* behind the teeth.

The sound made by this consonant must be pure and must not resemble the sound *sh*. Throughout this exercise the teeth remain clenched, the lips in the same open position and the tip of the tongue behind the incisors (100 times morning and evening if possible, the sound being produced loudly).

Exercise 3:

(a) Clear the throat forcefully.

(b) Clench the teeth with the lips wide open and whistle *ssa!* very loudly. 100 times to a beat of two: strike the thighs, strike the shoulders; for left-handed subjects, use the left hand only.

Exercise 4: The same exercise to bring the teeth together as in Exercise 2, but aimed to produce the voiced consonant:

$$ZZZ \text{ (100 Times)}$$

Pronounce the *z* as in *zeal*.

I should point out once more that the phonetic (spoken) consonant has not necessarily anything in common with the orthographic (written) consonant.

Exercise 5:

Articulate with volume and intensity *ga*, followed immediately by *ZA* (100 times, in the sitting position, giving alternate blows on the table and keeping sustained rhythm).

Exercise 6:

Practise the articulation of consonants in the strong position: *ssa za sse ze ssee zee sso zo ssoo zoo sswa zwa ssurn zurn sser zer sswee zwee* (20 times).

The articulation must be correct.

Exercise 7:

Same consonants in the weak position:
ass–az, ess–ez, eess–eez, oss–ooz, uss–uz, wass–waz, erss–erz, wees–weez (20 times).

Exercise 8:

Practise the same consonants in association with other phonetic sounds *(the s and the z must be correct)*:
atsa, aspi, pas, asp, rsa, abs, fsa, afs, zda, azd, bza, kssa, gzza, assk, agz (learn by heart and practise 20 times every day). In time with

the syllables, clasp and unclasp the hands: one syllable per movement.

Exercise 9: Practise the following words 25 times per day, articulating the sibilants with absolute correctness: *absurd, psalm, aspirin, aspro, psycho-analysis, instinctive, obsession, Rasputin, Assyrian, Esther, obstacle, St. Francis of Assisi, assumption, sturgeon, asphalt, assessor, examination, oxygen, ozone, suppression, Mazda, Absalom, abstinence, cosset, Esthonia, subsidiary, investiture, Istra, Isfahan, jasmine, Afghanistan, exaggeration.*

Exercise 10: Have the pupil articulate the titles of fables, poems, and stories, recording the result on tape:

EXAMPLES: *The Grasshopper and the Ant, The Labourer and his Children, The Wolf and the Stork, The Hound of the Baskervilles, The Merchant of Venice, Barchester Towers* etc. Practise each phrase 3 times.

Exercise 11: Subjects with a lisp automatically reveal it if made to count figures and numbers out aloud. It is valuable to practise counting from 1 to 100 and 100 to 1. Adults with a higher degree of culture frequently find a certain difficulty over this. The exercise of counting from 1 to 100 and 100 to 1 should be practised standing upright and should be divided up by the following movements, carried out in exact synchronization with the words:

arms: beat out bars of 2 time.
legs: alternate energetic taps with right and left leg.

Subjects should also be made to produce numbers with five, six or seven digits.

EXAMPLE: 67,625.

Articulate the whole number, then spell it out digit by digit forwards and backwards.

The defective consonants are found in those numbers including 6 or 7: 66,727; 16,765 etc.

Final exercise of the period

When the articulation has improved, each remedial session should be ended by an impromptu conversation on a subject related to the minor events and duties of everyday life.

If the subject uses his voice professionally: a priest, lawyer, doctor, teacher of any sort, professor, representative, salesman, this conversation should be oriented toward subjects of particular concern to the pupil: preaching, lawsuits, conversation with patients, lessons etc. The spheres in which the different professions are involved are vast and the remedial teacher must therefore familiarize himself with many aspects of life.

The systematic programme for a remedial session

1. Carry out briefly all the basic exercises, including those for the tongue, striking the front part of the bony palate several times with the tongue; imitation of the noise made by grooms with the tongue to encourage horses. Respiration exercises with the respirator are not to be forgotten.

Exercises for the nose and mouth

2. The pupil should be made to pay the very closest attention during all sessions, even those toward the end of the treatment, to the production of the sounds *se* and *ze*, whistling behind the clenched teeth, with the lips widely separated and without introducing the tip of the tongue behind the incisors. This is of vital importance.

3. A syllabic exercise, consisting of eight syllables, including consonants in the strong position.

4. A syllabic exercise, consisting of eight syllables, including consonants in the weak position (vary order).

5. An articulation exercise on words, phrases or numbers.

6. During the treatment impromptu conversations should be introduced on the spur of the moment.

This training, covering phonetics, respiration and psycho-motor co-ordination, may be of fairly long duration. The pupil should not be "passed out", until his cure is apparent during conversational speech, both for "live" voice and for tape recorded speech. It is, therefore, necessary that all trace of the lisp should be eliminated by the acquisition of automatically correct speech. Do not rest content with an "approximately" correct result.

ADULT DYSARTHRIA
SLURRING OF THE CONSONANTS

Slurring of the consonants and hissing are forms of dysarthria affecting the articulation of the fricative consonants *sh* and *zh* (as in pleasure).

For the correct production of these two sounds, the tongue rests against the lateral walls of the palate arch and against the upper molar sockets, thus allowing a wide passage for the escape of the current of air towards the funnel formed by the lips. If there are lateral gaps, air manages to escape between the edges of the tongue in the inner walls of the cheeks. The consonants *sh* and *zh* are then replaced by a mixed sound, which can be represented by the sound *shl.* Hissing is a similar defect, but in addition the rear part of the palatary velum, the base of the tongue and the muscles of the pharynx take part: the end result and the treatment of both disabilities is the same.

This slurring of the consonants is due to:

(a) Excessively pointed palate arch.
(b) A lateral gap in the dental arches.
(c) Maxillary atresia.
(d) Anomalous development of the incisor block.
(e) Under development of the lower jaw.
(f) Slight hearing defect.
(g) Faulty habits acquired in childhood.

The resulting dysfunction is sometimes accompanied by a slight facial paresis which entails a reduced motor activity of the maxillary muscles and of one cheek. A fair number of subjects with a "*hiss*" at the moment they articulate the consonants in question, give a sort of sideways twist to their mouth. Even the tongue is drawn in to participate in this movement and I have sometimes observed a "tic", involving the eyelids, which coincides with the effort to pronounce these sounds.

As in the case of the lisp we do not have to treat many adult cases of this type, except in cases of serious tonic stammering, which is sometimes complicated by a "hissing" defect.

The fricative consonants *sh* and *zh* are frequently confused popularly with the unvoiced and voiced sibilants *s* and *z*. During childhood parents find this form of dysarthria "sweet" or "amusing" and in naïve ignorance they imitate it.

EXAMPLES: "Mummy's little trezer" (treasure), "very shweet" or other errors which are, in effect, stupid and which can only result in an aggravation of the child's dysarthria.

The adult subject with a "hiss" is in fact not uncommon but he pays little heed except, I repeat, when this defect, carried over from his childhood, proves an impediment in his professional career.

REMEDIAL TREATMENT
EXERCISES

The "basic" exercises, designed to prepare the way for correction of phonetic defects, are even more important in the case of hissing defects than for other speech disorders. It is wrong to suppose that such remedial teaching will produce rapid results. It is especially difficult and months are required to obtain correct articulation and automatic auditory correction in the adult. As I have said many times, in all forms of phonetic remedial education instinctive auditory control, the adaptation of the ear to the new sound, takes a long time to achieve and requires energetic and sustained efforts.

Exercise 1: Carry out all the "basic"* exercises — for the maxilla and tongue, the drawing back of the upper lip, winking and release of the eyelids, "stuttering".

* "Basic" exercises are given in Chapter 1 on pages 6–9.

Throat clearing; exercises for the palatal velum, base of the tongue, exercises of the tongue and lips.

Exercise 2: Inflate and hollow the cheeks (20 times morning and evening).

Exercise 3: If there is any twisting of the mouth, practise 60 times the lateral projection of the lower jaw with the mouth wide open.

Exercise 4: Press the lips together. Move the whole muscular block of the lips as far as possible to the right and to the left (50 times per day). Keep the lips firmly closed throughout.

Exercise 5: Instruct the pupil:

    (a) To clench the teeth firmly together.
    (b) Push the lips well forward.
    (c) Blow the *sh* sound behind the teeth.

Practise the *shsh* sound 150 times per day at least.
Always blow the syllable out with force.

Exercise 6: When the pupil has successfully mastered the *sh* sound, practise in association with the sound *er* in the strong and weak position.

shshshsher   sher   ershshsh   ersh

The unvoiced consonant is fairly difficult to pronounce in the weak position (60 times morning and evening).

Exercise 7: When this unvoiced consonant has been mastered during the remedial sessions, the voiced *zh* (as in mea*s*ure) and the consonant sound *zhzhzh* should be practised in the same way: behind clenched teeth with the lips well forward.

Exercise 8: Associate the *zhzh* sound with *er:*

zhzhzher   zhzhzher (100 times)
erzhzh   erzhzh

Exercise 9: Introduce at this stage in the remedial treatment an attempt to produce these two consonants in association with all the vowels in the strong and weak positions:

shsha   ashsh   zha   azh

and in the same way with: *ay, ee, o, oo, wa, er, wee.*

10 times for all the syllables in the strong and weak positions. Learn these syllables by heart and practise them in the standing position with the hands beating out bars of 4 time and the legs bending then tapping on the floor.

Exercise 10: At this stage practise these sounds in the following words:

EXAMPLES: *ashen, encashment, shack, shear, shell, insure, treasure, leisure, measure, sheet, pleasure, shock, incision, parachute, hash, bunch, dish, shriek, unleash, Martian, marshal, sheen, shrill, crash, cashier, wish, revision, vision, shun, chiffon, shout.*

Exercise 11: Psycho-neural motor co-ordination:

(a) Stretch the right arm to the horizontal position.

(b) Strike the ground forcefully with the left foot.

(c) Raise the left arm above the head.

(d) Lower the right arm.

(e) Strike the ground forcefully with the right foot.

(f) Lower the left arm.

In perfect synchronization with these movements, articulate short phrases, constructed to contain words with these two consonants (one syllable per movement).

EXAMPLES: *He shouted with pleasure at the show.*
He made sure of the revision of the third sheet.
The publisher shunned every pleasure.
She wore beige chiffon.
Measure for measure diverts a man's leisure.

Exercise 12: The following exercise which the pupil must practise assiduously at home permits the muscular and motor differentiation of these fricative consonants and the sibilants:

sha	clench the teeth	*ja(zha)*
pout the lips forwards		pout the lips forwards
sa	clench the teeth	*za*
open the lips		open the lips

Working in front of the mirror gives good results in this case.

In case of maxillary malformation, defective seating of the teeth, gaps in the dental arches, defective maxillo-facial balance, a qualified mouth specialist must be brought in.

For the sequence of a remedial session of this type, use the example given for lisping.*

It must never be forgotten that the aim of this remedial treatment is to instil the reflex, the automatic performance of the corrected action. We eliminate a bad habit, replacing it by a positive one. Was it not Watson who said: "The conditioned reflex is the basic unit, which is multiplied into habit".

THE CONFUSION OR FAULTY ARTICULATION OF PHONETIC SOUNDS ALTERATIONS IN VOCAL TIMBRE

Astonishing as it may seem I have often found the same speech defects in adults as in children. These are the people who were backward in speaking in early life, who, neglected by their families, are sometimes unaware of their disabilities.

During the ten years that I was responsible at the Conservatoire National de Musique for the course in "Applied Phonetics for Singers", I met young people who confused the guttural and dental consonants (*mekro* for *metro*) (*crain* for *train*), or who had never managed to pronounce the lateral *l* and replaced it with an *n*. Such pupils were quite astonished and disturbed when their faults were

* Lisping: Chapter IX page 119 *et seq.*

brought home to them. They had had no suspicions. The disability was to some degree extended to their orthography, where, in dictation, they confused the voiced and unvoiced consonants, writing *p* for *b*, *z* for *sh*, *d* for *t*, and *m* for *n*. As for the lingual dorsal *r*, required in the course of singing, it was out of the question for them. Months of exercises were required to obtain even a clumsy representation of this, unless such young people happened to come from an area of the provinces where the local accent still includes the lingual dorsal *r* which they are accustomed to incorporate in their speech. The vowels are also distorted and lose their tonal quality. Such defects which are found especially in the case of illiterates, require a course of remedial treatment "tailored" to their requirements.

Exercise 1: Production of the *l* by exercises designed to stimulate the activity of the three parts of the tongue:

the base   the rear   the tip (ka! ya! da! sa!)

Rapid vibrations of the tip of the tongue on the lips (outside), starting with a plosive labial consonant:

ba! lalalalala (10 times) and of course basic exercises.

Exercise 2: Trace the subject's confused consonants, writing them down on the board. Read them:

(a) from the board
(b) from the lips of the teacher
(c) articulate them correctly.

The teacher should verify that the pharynx is being used for the articulation of the voiced sounds, placing his hands on the pupil's thyroid cartilage and on his own.

Exercise 3: Clearing the throat deep down is an efficient aid in the correction of the confused guttural and dental consonants.

EXAMPLE: *Ka*, immediately followed by *ta* (with the teeth immediately opposite each other). In this case also reading from the board, reading from the lips of the teacher and articulation should be practised (40 times).

Exercise 4: Practise the dentals *d* and *t* in association with the *r*, *tra, dra.*

To start with, the two sounds must be practised separately.

The correct automatic articulation of single syllables should then be mastered, the one following the other in quick succession *tera dera* (100 times).

Exercise 5: To make sure of the correct pronunciation of these sounds, practise them with the gutturals: *kra gra* (100 times with no errors).

Exercise 6: Repeat in association with all the vowels: *ay, ee, o, oo, wa, er, wee.*

Exercise 7: If the timbre of the vowels is distorted, practise the defective vowels individually. In general the long *ah* (as in *large*) is pronounced badly.

Exercise 8: Once the sounds are articulated without being confused they should be incorporated in all words, which have of course been produced to include the correctly articulated consonants.

EXAMPLES: *attraction, troll, temperament, loiter, minority, balloon, illumination, parabola, traverse, attribute, polarization, polychrome, milk, Memnon.*

Exercise 9: Construct phrases including the words given above or similar words and articulate them in time with bars of 6 time, beaten out with both hands:

1	2	3
Strike the knees	the knees	the knees
4	5	6
Strike the shoulders	the shoulders	the shoulders

EXAMPLES: Fol de rol, I'm a troll,
Fol de rol, sang the troll.
Memnon was slain in far distant Troy.
The rocket traversed the sky in parabola.

It is clear how easy it is for teacher and pupil to find large numbers of new phrases to practise everyday, both impromptu and learnt. The impromptu work is preferable owing to the vital importance of developing the imagination.

Exercise 10: As soon as the improvement appears beyond doubt, make the subject conduct short conversations every day on subjects of interest to him. They should from time to time be recorded on tape.

As regards the sequence of the remedial session, follow the indications given for lisping.*

* Lisping: Chapter IX page 179 *et seq.*

CHAPTER X

ADULT APHASIAS

To CREATE the power of speech in the child. To restore the power of speech to the adult. Two related yet quite dissimilar spheres of remedial work. I believe the first to be easier to accomplish and fraught with less disappointment.

Let me begin with a few definitions.

Aphasia is the loss by the memory of those symbols which man employs to communicate with his like. The organs of speech are quite normal; the inhibitive lesion lies in the brain. The Broca motor aphasia is the name given to the loss of the movements of articulation, and the Wernicke sensory aphasia to the inability to understand the spoken language (auditory aphasia or word deafness) and the written language (alexia or word blindness), where neither the mechanisms of hearing nor sight are affected. In a word aphasia describes the state of having forgotten the meaning of language in all its forms: read, heard, written or spoken.

The patient with a Broca motor aphasia understands what is said to him, but cannot reply, repeat what has been said or speak. It is the sensory motor memory and the sensory motor mechanisms of language that are affected. Gestures are forgotten, there is apraxia or motor amnesia, but the power of movement is still there. Apraxia comprises the loss of the knowledge how to speak, the loss of the technique of the spoken word.

The patient with a Wernicke sensory aphasia does not understand what is said to him, but he can speak. He perceives speech only as a noise of which he cannot grasp the significance; he is like a traveller in a foreign land, who cannot understand what is said to him. The Wernicke aphasia is localized in the rear sector of the left temporo-parietal lobe, the so-called Wernicke area.

Agraphia is to the written language what aphasia is to the spoken language.

Pure motor aphasia, without loss of the ability to understand speech, reading and writing, is an oro-laryngeal anarthria or apraxia, which is localized at the base of the third frontal convolution. The classical name for anarthria is aphemia. Motor aphasia, however, is most frequently found in conjunction with sensory aphasia and the combination of these two aphasias constitutes the form most usually found. The term aphasia, pure and simple, is the most convenient description, although in fact it covers two classes of symptoms.

Aphasia is always accompanied by a serious deficiency in the intellectual sphere. The inner language — of which speech and the written word are merely translations — is profoundly affected. As a result the external language becomes inhibited. Aphasia brings together various different classes of symptom, the connection between which is the result of anatomical contiguity in the brain: ideo-motor apraxia (anarthria and agraphia); auditory aphasia (word deafness) and visual aphasia (word blindness); memory breakdown (motor amnesia and sensory amnesia); defective inner language, regression of the function of thought and a deficiency in the higher processes of abstraction.

In those aphasic cases which are accessible to remedial treatment, i.e. the less serious and more recent cases, the patient makes great efforts to speak. He at least understands in part and with certain delay what is said to him. He carries out the orders he is given, for example; open your mouth, shut your eyes, raise your hand. Very often he can only carry out the first instruction and goes on repeating the same gesture instead of the following ones. Of course, if the proof of the acceptance of orders is to have any value, one must avoid at all costs supplementing the word of mouth with an indicative gesture. The family tend to believe that the patient understands everything because they use the language of gestures to the maximum.

Often the patient is capable of naming various objects which are pointed out to him, although he does so slowly and with some distortion of word structure. The vocabulary is very limited; the language almost that of pidgin English, without pronouns, conjunctions or any connecting words (syntax is lacking). A few interjections and indiscriminate sounds, however, survive the chaos. Gestures are numerous and inappropriate. Repetition always predominates over spontaneous utterance. Automatism in speech generally survives well and the patient is able to say "Our Father" and count from one to twenty on his fingers.

Some aphasic patients are very loquacious but their ideas are disconnected; they are mentally disorganized as a result of defective function of the higher psychic centres. Attention, memory and the association of ideas are lacking. The same disability is apparent in the motor sphere; they have lost control of their gestures; in other words the aphasia affects both ideation and motor function. They often use quite inappropriate words or invent new ones; this disorder is known as paraphrasia. In the next stage of this disorder, the patient creates his own system of articulation, which is almost correct, but completely incomprehensible; this form of aphasia is known by the name of jargonism.

In general aphasic patients placed in our care are presumed to be mentally capable of reading, but it is difficult to check their reading potential and one often gains the impression that their potential is far more limited than either they or their family suspect.

If they write it is usually with the left hand and in pencil. The characters are unformed. They try very hard with very little to show for it, whether they are taking dictation or copying. The same difficulty, the same mistakes occur in their attempts at arithmetic; the complexity of the effort required is too much for the subject who can no longer act mechanically, and brings him to a stop. The musical sense is altered, although some aphasic patients manage to sing simple tunes in which occasional words or parts of phrases emerge more or less correctly pronounced. The movements of the lips and tongue are markedly clumsy which is only natural in a disorder of this type. The emotional behaviour of such patients is normally exaggerated; they are easily moved, weep, complain of the difficulty they find in speaking and welcome the teacher with transports of joy. Sometimes the origin of such disorders can be traced to cranial injury (damage to the parieto-occipital region of the left hemisphere).

In the treatment of aphasia there is some chance of success, provided the aphasia is of recent origin (3 to 4 months), if the subject is still young (40 to 50 years old), if the intellectual deficiency is not too marked, if he appears to understand at any rate part of what is said, if the motor lesions (hemiplegia) have already receded, and finally if his inner language appears to be intact.

LANGUAGE DISORDERS
REMEDIAL EDUCATION

The teacher's first duty is to get a clear picture of the state of his patient's verbal and intellectual functions.

1. Verbal functions. An assessment must be made of his defects of articulation, vocabulary and syntax.

Those subjects who are placed in our care are normally not anarthrics (i.e. real cases of speech loss), but dysarthrics (i.e. cases of loss of speech as a result of distortion, confusion or word mutilation). The vocabulary is either forgotten or disturbed by the endless repetition of the same words or made incomprehensible by the substitution of words or the distortion of words (paraphrasia). All trace of syntax vanishes; the subject speaks a sort of pidgin English; the discipline of grammar disappears and often we get jargonism, logorrhoea and verbal confusion. The teacher will attach great importance to the test of whether his orders are understood, which is a good method of assessing the word deafness of the patient; starting with simple orders, we work up to more and more complicated orders, e.g. "Open the door", "Give me your right hand", "Please look at the time", etc.

The written language should be checked in the same way. Is the patient suffering from alexia, i.e. verbal blindness, either in respect of letters, words or phrases? The texts, placed before him, include orders and the test is whether he obeys them. Writing defects (agraphia) are then investigated, whether in composition, dictation or copying. Often the patient suffers from paragraphia, i.e. his words are deformed or confused.

It is essential for the remedial teacher to attempt to form an approximate assessment of the intellectual condition of the patient; he must take into account the patient's attention, judgement, reasoning, memory and arithmetical capacity. As regards memory, the lost vocabulary is already a sign of deficiency. As Jean Delay has advised, we then examine whether the didactic and affective memory has been affected; the didactic memory concerns the events of his life. The affective memory is often better retained than the didactic.

The patient has often lost the power of calculating: he cannot carry out the simplest arithmetical operations, let alone financial calculations. His powers of attention are easily exhausted, whereas his judgement remains relatively unimpaired.

This assessment of the patient's condition is completed by looking for any signs of spatial disorientation: confusion of left and right. In everyday life the victim of aphasia cannot find his way about the town. His chronological orientation is equally affected: he cannot read the time or set his watch by a clock.

It is easy to see that the less disturbance there is of his intellectual functions, the more chance our exercises have of success. The sequence to be followed is first to develop and regulate the breathing by methodical spiroscopic exercises and by the daily practice of the basic exercises. At the same time as these exercises, which are designed to develop suppleness, a systematic effort must be made to alleviate the mutism on the lines of the treatment for retarded speech and deafness in children. Then if, as is normally the case, the patient has retained a few words, these should be used in the attempt to recover the ground that has been lost. To this end it is a good thing to work in front of the mirror, then make the subject imitate the movements of articulation carried out close to him. The phonetic sounds which he has retained are used to produce associated sounds, sometimes with the aid of lip-reading.

At the same time the patient should be made to feel the laryngeal vibrations which accompany the vocal sounds. We attempt to mobilize the powers of hearing, sight, touch and attention and at the same time to provoke the action of the glottis, i.e. the initial speech sound.

To complete these first attempts to secure the imitation of the movements of speech, lip reading and movement of the glottis, we undertake gymnastic exercises for the speech organs, starting with the training of the tongue: upward and downward movements, withdrawing and extending forwards, upwards, to the right, to the left and downwards. After this we deal with the motor function of the lower jaw (opening, closing and lateral movements).

If satisfactory results are achieved during the initial sessions, attention is then directed to developing the mobility of the lips and cheeks in connection with the action of the tongue and lower jaw.

All these exercises are easier to describe than to carry out, since obstacles rise up at every moment, sometimes proving insurmountable where the directing centres of the brain refuse to undertake again their function of neuro-motor control. This all depends on the extent and depth of the lesions, the activation of supplementary action by the cortex and the energy of the subject and his family. The latter have in fact an important part to play, since the exercises must be carried on at home.

I must stress that attempts at the recovery of speech, and the ability to read and write must be made simultaneously; never try to activate these functions separately. One should use a complementary auditory and graphic effect, i.e. present the patient with the written word, pronouncing it at the same time. When he has repeated it, make him write it down. Unless this technique is followed, there is a risk that the treatment will not achieve the results anticipated.

In favourable cases the aphasic patient gradually regains the use of the mechanisms for the emission and articulation of the spoken word; his power of automatic association is restored; his aphasia, his amnesia, his apraxia are to some extent eliminated.

Recovery is not complete, but a part of his functions is regained and his burden is lightened.

APHASIA AND APHONIA AS A
RESULT OF SHOCK

These disorders are especially accessible to remedial treatment since they are not the result of organic lesions. They are due only to disordered motor co-ordination of the muscles of speech and respiration, provoked by a traumatic short-circuit. Only remedial education is capable of curing these functional disorders, both from the point of view of speech and of respiration. The marked contractions of the cervical muscles, the uncontrolled efforts, which serve no useful purpose, indicate the inadequacy of the supply of air which generates the vocal sound. The patient tries in vain to find his voice. He can only do so after normal respiration has been restored and the exaggerated expenditure of unprofitable energy, in which he indulges, eliminated.

Under the influence of respiration exercises the contractions give way. Functional co-ordination is restored; the shortness of breath and the contractions of the muscles which were impeding the emission of vocal sound disappear, once the harmony of the act of respiration has been restored. It is then time to make attempts at speech. This is the second stage of the remedial treatment and is decisive although difficult to accomplish.

The position of the larynx is of capital importance. The patient has a tendency to raise the vocal organ too high. This must therefore be lowered by a steady pressure on the thyroid plate from above downwards and by bringing the chin down toward the area of the chest. By dipping the thyroid we remove some of the tension from the thyro-arytenoid muscles and in consequence the vocal cords are generally relaxed.

An attempt should then be made to articulate the vowels with, as far as possible, a spontaneous unforced emission of sound. As soon as this first step has been taken the pupil should be made to draw out the sound and should be taught several very simple exercises in vocal rhythm and modulation. This phonetic training leads up unobtrusively to articulation, i.e. toward the cure of the condition. It is enough to put the patient on the right road to speech for him to get his bearings and move steadily toward proper phonation.

It is often of advantage to make the patient deaf by artificial means so that he loses acoustic control of his defects; his voice, though sub-normal, is recovered and when the artificial deafness is then abruptly eliminated, he perceives that his voice is once more audible. No patient ever suffers from a mild aphasia or one that falls within restricted limits. Some put up a facade, but all are seriously affected; there are few aspects of remedial treatment that require greater efforts or more patience and self-sacrifice. The remedial process is one of careful diagnosis and involves the use of a wide variety of techniques, of imagination and intuition, in order to seize the vital opportunity.

The most difficult patients to treat are those who tirelessly repeat the same word, with all the shades of intonation and modulation normally present in the voice. One of my patients used to articulate the word "today". He imparted a tone either amiable or angry to this, the sole expression in his vocabulary. Another patient (a woman) was accustomed to say "No", "No", for seconds, minutes, hours or for the whole day. The negative particle served to express her impressions, feelings or her anger. This phonetic "tic" has to be eliminated by remedial education; it must be forgotten, not an easy task, since the parasitic word is recalcitrant and is used by the patient with every accent of the mind, the emotions and the personality. Psychotherapy, it should be realized, represents only one half of the technique of remedial education. The patient himself and the "family" must play their part. The role of the "family" is really extended to cover eight or nine entities: wife or husband, children, uncles, aunts, cousins, friends, tradesmen, porters, employees ... Everyone has his say, puts in his word and complicates the task of the person in charge of remedial education. The teacher must stand firm as a rock against the swirling waves and tides of this sea of emotion. We must "hold on" and try to restrict the reporting of collective views, whether favourable or not, to a spell of three or four minutes during each session.

I can only give an approximate idea of the sequence of a remedial session for aphasic patients. It will serve as a model of the exercises to be practised, but it must be understood that the task of the remedial worker is to vary and adapt the programme of each period, to suit the physical and psychic state of the patient from day to day. Such patients can be so interesting, so pitiful, so unhappy.

EXERCISES

Exercise 1: The "basic" exercises are vital since the patient is often no longer aware of the mechanisms of phonation and articulation. He must be helped to re-adapt to perform these functions, but it is at the same time important to regulate the amount of training given in order to suit the patient's capacity.

(a) The lowering and energetic raising of the maxilla must be carried out at least four times per day.

(b) The patient's right arm is often paralysed. He should be taught to use his left to set the pace and beat time for his attempts at phonation. He should try to count aloud to the beat of two, three and four time.

Exercise 2: Make the patient raise his good hand, or, if neither are paralyzed, both hands to the level of his face. Instruct him to "cover" and "uncover" his face, saying at the same time "cover" and "uncover" (30 times).

Exercise 3: In three time:

(a) Open the mouth
(b) Put out the tongue
(c) Close the mouth
(20 times).

Exercise 4: In two time (striking the thigh and the shoulder):

(a) Close the lips tightly together.
(b) Explode sharply the labial plosive syllables *ba* or *pa*.

If the patient obeys this, make him associate these consonants with all the vowels. Watch for distortion, as the patient will have forgotten the feel of vocal timbre:

*ay–ee–o(*pot*)–oo–wa–er*

Repeat as often as possible without tiring the patient.

Exercise 5: Practise all the consonants. Articulation of the consonants is difficult to restore, since in nine cases out of ten the patient has completely forgotten how to articulate. The mechanism must therefore be re-learnt in the following sequence:

ka–ga   The beginning of the movement is indicated by clearing the throat, if the patient is able to accomplish this. If he cannot, the method of articulation can be brought home to him by the teacher placing his hand on the patient's throat.

da–ta–na Clench the teeth and allow the two consonants to burst out; the *na* is produced more softly. If necessary the patient should be made to bite the tip of his tongue very gently in order to exteriorize the consonant and make it more comprehensible.

zha–sha   Clench the teeth, pouting the lips to blow out the *sh*, then the *zh* behind the incisors.

sa–za   Clench the teeth, open the lips. Blow softly behind the teeth.

l   Vibrations of the tip of the tongue on the outside of the lips.

fa–va   Bite the lower lip. Blow out the *fff* and *vvvvvvv*

the two *x* (Voiced and unvoiced as in "exit" and "excess".) Where possible make the patient practise *Kehssa–gza (kssagza).*

ma   Press the patient's hand gently *m...m...m.*

ya   Make a small gap between the back of the tongue and the bony palate and practise *eeleeaeella...*

As soon as each consonant has been restored, it should be practised with all the vowels.

Exercise 6: Instruct the patient to indicate with the left hand:

The top of his head.	The left elbow.
The nape of the neck.	The thumbs.
The forehead.	The left shoulder.
The right ear.	The little fingers.
The left eye.	The right shoulder.
The neck (front).	The third fingers.
The left ear.	The palms of the hands.
The right eye.	The right knee.
The chest.	The back of the hands.
The back.	The left knee.
The thighs.	The right foot.
The right shoulder.	The left foot.

Exercise 7: The patient is ordered to carry out different movements. This exercise has one aim alone: "to reactivate the cerebral and motor control mechanisms which have been disturbed or suppressed".

(a) Raise the left shoulder. Lower it.

The direction for these movements should be given one after the other.

(b) Close the left eye. Open it.

(c) Raise both shoulders. Lower them.

Do not repeat this for each shoulder individually.

(d) Close the right eye. Open it.

(e) Tap on the floor with the left foot.

(f) Write (in pencil) your name and address.

(g) Spell and read what you have written.

(h) Place your hand on the table.

(i) Separate your fingers; bring them together again.

Exercise 8: According to the profession previously exercised by the aphasic patient, help him to recollect matters relating to that profession:

(a) By words which are associated with the appropriate ideas.

(b) By phrases, constructed from such words and ideas.

(c) By questions on the selected subject: help the patient to answer.

EXAMPLE: Let us imagine that the patient was connected with the provision trade (grocery):

(a) Quote the names of his employees (if he had several).

(b) Make him try to describe the position of the cash register. (pronouncing the word "cash") in the shop.

(c) Use the words "biscuits", "jam".

(d) Treat the word "coffee" in the same way, getting the patient to name different makes. Take advantage of this to practise association of ideas: When do we drink coffee? What do we put in it? And, if possible, relate to the patient the history of the consumption of coffee.

(e) Make the pupil enumerate the names of the goods for the purchase and sale of which he was responsible.

EXAMPLES: rice, oil, salt, condiments, dried vegetables, dairy produce, etc.

It is a good thing to make the patient write down the words he has produced. They can then be read over a few minutes later and the sense explained again. This exercise is obviously only an example. It could easily be adapted to any of the liberal professions or manual crafts. I have used this technique to treat politicians, administrators, engineers, etc.

Exercise 9: It is advisable to start each session with exercises on syllables using related consonants together with vowels.

EXAMPLES: *babri–codra* (adult aphasic patients, like children, mix gutturals and dentals and read: *totlate* for *chocolate*, *pottle* for *bottle*, *Mecropole* for *Metropole* etc.) *crater, cricri, fraga, prader, flo–fru–vra–kssa–gzou–sla–tra–dray*.

Always persevere with the defective syllables, without however arousing his obstinacy. One must "tack" to and fro between the sounds, which have become distorted or have disappeared.

Exercise 10: In the frequent case where the aphasic patient uses one word for another, e. g. where he says "salad" when confronted with the word "bottle", it is useful to use the former word as a starting point.

EXAMPLE: In the above case the patient may then be asked to write down the names of the salads he knows and indicate the place of the salad in a meal and the sort of dish it is served in. How is it dressed? The patient may be asked to try to remember a particular form of salad dressing, or he may be asked about "vinegar". Thus by association of ideas we progress to wine and from wine to bottle, etc. Ideas must always be linked together in our development of judgement and memory.

The subject of food was chosen deliberately. I have noticed that aphasic patients, even the most cultured, are always interested in gastronomic matters, possibly due to their preoccupation with the diets imposed on them by the doctors. This method of training can easily be switched to the arts, to literature or to any other subject capable of activating the memory, stimulating the attention and restoring speech to patients suffering from aphasia of varying degrees of severity.

Exercise 11: We must use caution in dealing with aphemic patients: a hemiplegic patient's general motor functions may show an improvement and he may present an almost normal picture, and then suddenly, influenced by some unknown psychic factor, there are symptoms of obvious cerebral disorder. There is no need to become upset about this, one must simply retrace one's steps and for several periods practise the initial exercises. Never omit the psycho-neural motor movements.

Make the patient go through the conjugation of verbs orally 9 or 10 times.

EXAMPLE: "I walk slowly forward" (normal walk). "I walk quickly backwards", suiting the action to the words, provided of course that the general motor functions permit this to be done.

It can be seen that everything connected with the remedial education of adult aphasic patients must be delicately and rightly handled. We have to show both toward the patient and his circle, imagination, great patience and devotion to the task. It is equally important to be able to make contact with the patient.

CHAPTER XI

LACK OF PSYCHO-NEURAL MOTOR CO-ORDINATION IN THE ADULT

STAMMERING, STUTTERING, ARRHYTHMIC DISORDERS AND INHIBITION

It is difficult to imagine any language defect that afflicts the victim with a more obsessive, anguished anxiety or fetters him in deeper torment than severe tonic stammering. Dissatisfied with themselves, fettered and bound with inner knots, such patients bear a grudge against life, against their families and against those who are treating them, when, in spite of all the effort spent, all the practice and all the expense of will-power, the treatment does not prove as effective as they had hoped.

Remedial treatment, whatever the type, is always of long duration. Very often its results are in inverse proportion to the level of intelligence of the patient. The more cultured the stammering patient, the more he thinks, the more he studies his infirmity (for that is what it is), and the more critical he is of the exercises which he is advised to carry out; the greater the deterioration in his psycho-nervous state, the less the progress he makes. His distress is the greater for the fact that when he is alone, in a calm state, far from any questioner, he can converse with ease and can even make eloquent speeches.

Then in certain cases, under certain conditions, certain circumstances, he appears to be cured, only to relapse into his former state at the first opportunity. The essence of "stammering" is its episodic nature, and this is what astonishes the family and indeed the patient himself. How often have I heard it said: "It's a strange thing; but he doesn't stammer all the time; it comes in fits and starts". But unfortunately these stammering fits occur often and at the most inopportune moments.

Stammering is not a speech defect, it is a functional disorder of the neuro-cerebral psycho-motor mechanisms; it is the outstanding symptom of a complex disability. It is an obvious source of embarrassment. The patient stumbles over the spoken word, just as a patient suffering from vertigo falls over when he attempts to stand upright. Inability to speak is distressing for the patient who has lost his voice, the aphasic victim or the laryngectomy patient, but I believe that for the stammering patient, who "could speak", it is even more painful, more brutal, more intolerable in the literal sense of that word. The adult stammerer is only the continuation of a stammering child who has not been treated. Having already studied the causes of the stammer in children, I shall not go over them again.

My sole aim is to reveal clearly the agony suffered by the stammerer. As a rule this is not known or is misunderstood, but it is a problem familiar to me... With all my heart, all my strength, all my knowledge I wish to relieve this agony.

The victim of a severe tonic stammer is in the grip of a constant struggle between ideation and its immediate expression: the spoken word. Respiratory disorder is a frequent symptom and the fear of speaking, and a feeling of intense anxiety at having to do so, dominate the life of the stammering patient. The emotion makes its influence felt on all the important physiological systems of the body. In regard to respiration, this is felt as an increase in the respiratory rhythm, even to the extent of panting. This can only aggravate the malfunction of the diaphragm. The movements of the diaphragm cannot effect expiration, capable of producing speech, any more than fibrillation of the heart can ensure the correct circulation of the blood; one could by analogy almost speak of "diaphragmatic fibrillation".* It should be noted that stammering is perhaps a little less common among women than among men although I have frequently seen cases of female tonic

* Dr. Chazal. *Le Bégaiement* (Stammering) January 1961.

stammering. Research is at present being carried out on stammering. A system based on auditory methods has been put into use for remedial treatment. In reality nothing can be effective which does not act on the main physiological systems of the body. This psycho-neural motor defect stems from a frustrated left-hand tendency, disordered respiration, general motor construction, marked inhibition, hyperaffectivity, disturbed psychic function and an involuntary contraction of the pharynx and larynx. As regards techniques of remedial treatment, everyone has his own methods which he believes the best. This is wrong. Stammering in all its multiple aspects is only amenable to multisensory remedial treatment. Corrective exercises must be designed specially to suit each individual case.

The stammering subject must receive individual treatment. Treatment may prove successful for one patient, but not for others. There is no universal panacea for this disorder. The first thing is to reassure the subject, inspire him with confidence and at each session give him a new influx of energy.

The range of psychic and personality states displayed by a serious case of stammering is so wide as to defy the imagination. All this aggravates the task of the teacher. Optimism is rare among stammering subjects. We have to meet their fits of depression, like their fits of enthusiasm, with an indefatigable display of will-power, with indulgent firmness, a supple and alert imagination and complete devotion to the task. I do not claim that our techniques are universally efficacious; we often meet with checks, failures too, and our successes are sometimes only temporary. In this type of remedial treatment, therefore, one should never promise a complete cure; but everything should be done to achieve it.

I give below a series of exercises which have often given positive beneficial results. They are of varied application. It must never be forgotten, however, that the success of remedial treatment depends on the teacher, the pupil and the pupil's circle. I have, moreover, been able to record during my professional career a number of cures, and cures of lasting duration. My sincere good wishes go to those who will apply the techniques indicated, so that they may free those who suffer so gravely from stammering from their distressing bonds.

RESPIRATION EXERCISES

The types of respiration in the male and female are: male — abdomen and diaphragm; female — upper costal.

Since controlled respiration is the cornerstone of remedial treatment, the stammering patient must be trained to develop the "enlarged" respiration, used by the professional singer. The stammerer (of either sex) must, like the professional singer, develop a slow, deep and regular movement of expiration.

Exercise 1: Lying down (on a hard, resistant surface), breathe in through the nostrils (without exaggerated sniffing). The thoracic cage and the abdominal cavity should be dilated in a single movement.

Expiration: the abdominal cavity is progressively and very slowly retracted. The thoracic cage gradually falls. Breathe out slowly through the mouth (20 times morning and evening).

Exercise 2: Same exercise as before with the addition of a whispered count of 1 to 20–25, 30 or more, in place of the silent expiration.

The pupil should be recommended to practise these exercises at home morning and evening (20 times).

Exercise 3: Sitting position:

Respiration exercise, using the Respirator.

Nasal respiration: 3 minutes for each nostril.

Buccal respiration: a minimum of 10 minutes per day.

Exercise 4: Respiration in the upright (standing) position:

Same respiratory exercises as those carried out in the lying position. The pupil stands very straight with the arms lowered.

Inspiration: rapid, deep and silent breathing (through the nostrils) without sniffing and without raising the shoulders.

Expiration: slow, very slow, breathing out through the mouth with gradual retraction of the muscles of the abdominal band (15 times morning and evening).

Exercise 5: Upright position. Same exercise as before but, in place of the silent expiration, articulate the following phrase in a low voice: "I must breathe out slowly and deeply".

This phrase should be repeated as often as possible without breathing in. Three or four times at least or more, according to standard of training (practise 6 times daily).

Exercise 6: Final respiratory exercise, carried out in the upright position. Breathe in and out rapidly, deeply, and silently twenty times, blowing energetically as if to extinguish a candle in one go.

Co-ordination exercises in the sitting position

Exercise 1: Learn by heart forwards and backwards, our series of syllables: *ba–bay–bo* (as in *pot*)–*boo–bee–bor–ber–bwa–bwee* from the first to the ninth and the ninth to the first (without a mistake).

Then this same series of vowels with each of the following consonants:

k–d–f–g–j–sh–l–m–n–p–r–s–t–v–x(ks)–y–z.

Exercise 2: With the hands laid flat on the table, the fingers are raised and lowered in time with the above syllables, which have been learnt by heart.

Imitate five finger exercises on the piano: thumb, index finger, second, third and fourth fingers, then in reverse order back to the thumb. Four times per day for these series of syllables.

This exercise may give the stammerer the rhythm in speech which he requires in his everyday life.

Exercise 3: All the basic exercises. The pupil should never be permitted to omit them. It is easy to see that the restoration of suppleness to the organs and muscles of phonation and articulation assumes a capital importance in the remedial treatment of cases of stammering. Clearing of the throat well at the back must not be forgotten.

Exercise 4: Non-differentiated articulation should be practised in conjunction with the puppet exercises. Dr. Chazal has stated that for the frustrated left-hander (a great many stammering cases are in fact left-handers, who have suffered from ignorant attempts to make them right-handed) the puppet exercise is of great value. At the start of the training, the left hand is a "poor follower" of the right. After a period of practice of varying duration, it picks up a satisfactory rhythm again and may then surpass the right hand in rapidity of movement.

Exercise 5: The stammering subject is made to count out beats of 2, 3, 4, 5 and 6 time successively and then in descending order back to a beat of 2.

Exercise 6: The pupil is then instructed to pronounce, in time with each beat, any syllable that comes into his head, in no established order and without the syllables forming words.

EXAMPLE: *tree soo na plo gar shee mee stroo na pwee bwee pwa kass ploo* etc. The time should be fairly fast: $^1/_4$ second per beat.

This is a difficult exercise for the pupil to carry out. It is, however, excellent training and must be persevered with. It is even possible to get the subject to the stage of pronouncing two or three syllables per beat. It also provides a very valuable exercise for rhythm. It requires a great deal of patience on the part of the teacher and effort on the part of the pupil.

A tape recording is of great use in this exercise.

Exercise 7: Strike the table with the hands and then turn them over. Strike again, saying each time (the first syllable of the words in exact time with the movements):

"Flat position" (palm of the hands on the table).

"Reverse position" (palms upturned).

Practise this exercise 25 times.

Exercise 8: The pupil should be taught the importance of the "stress" in the spoken language.

The "stress" is a phonetic figure, marked by a definite accentuation. This accent must be felt, since it is based only on rhythm. It is the stress that ensures the rhythm and harmonious balance of the division of phrases in the sentence. There are certain units of time which are of fundamental importance both for our physical movements, walking for example, and for the grouping or classification of our sense perceptions, and which are intimately linked with the functions, controlling the whole organism: the beat of the pulse and the respiration. The spoken language stands in equal need of this grouping or sub-division of time periods and intuitively repeats certain stresses. Just as in "plain song", the accents, required by the normal reading of a text, provide a sort of measure of time, when they are given rhythmic accentuated stress and placed at equal distances from each other.

Examples of "stresses":

> Rhythm: is vertical
> Beat: is horizontal   4 stresses

A single word or syllable can alone constitute a stress.

EXAMPLE:

Alas
Why is it
the doctors decide   (5 stresses)
so late
for re-education?

It is not always easy to familiarize the stammering subject with the rhythmic balancing of stress, but it can be done.

Give the pupil a word, on which to build up a sentence. He then allots the stresses.

EXAMPLE: Suggest the word "discover". Vasco da Gama: the Portuguese explorer: sailed round: the Cape of Good Hope: to discover India (5 stresses).

Obviously we have to take account of the age, level of culture, intelligence and psychic background of the patient in order to adapt the themes skilfully, so as to stimulate his imagination.

Exercise 9: Once the principle of the stress has been assimilated, the pupil is made to read or recite texts, emphasizing, by means of bodily movements, the rhythmic balance of the spoken language.

EXAMPLE: Swing the arms in a circular direction with the spoken stress coinciding with the start of each circular movement. In this case the duration of the stress must be adapted individually to the tempo of the movements. The stresses may also be balanced to coincide with the striking of the hands on the knees or the table alternately. If he is able to carry out these exercises properly, he should practise them at home also.

EXERCISES IN THE UPRIGHT POSITION

For these exercises refer to the chapter on the remedial education of children who suffer from stammering.
Add the following:

Exercise 1:

Upper limbs	Use the left hand to count out a beat in six time — three beats up, three beats down. Carry out the following movements with the right hand: Stretch out in the horizontal position; Clench the fist; Open the hand; Strike the knee twice. The sixth beat is not indicated by any movement, the hand remains stationary on the knee.
Lower limbs	Strike three taps with the right foot; Strike three taps with the left foot.

These dissociated movements must be exactly synchronized.

In time with the movements, keeping perfect rhythm, enumerate 12 nouns:

of geographic connection
of historic connection
of mathematical connection etc.

Practise ten times by heart in the original order, then in reverse order.

and of professional concern to the stammering or stuttering subject, victim of arrhythmia or inhibition. Remedial treatment is similar in kind for all disorders; it is, however, varied in the extent of its application to suit the seriousness of the defect.

Exercise 2:

(a) Lean well forward, arms stretched straight backwards.
(b) Lean over as far as possible backwards with the arms outstretched forwards.
(c) Back to normal position, arms by the sides.
(d) Raise the arms above the head.
(e) Bring the arms down to the level of the face (palms downward).
(f) Separate the fingers.
(g) Bring the fingers together.
(h) Clench the fists.
(i) Open the hands.

In time with the execution of these nine movements, articulate by heart the names of the nine Muses and their attributes.

Clio:	Muse of History	As usual from first to
Euterpe:	Muse of Music	last and then from last
Terpsichore:	Muse of Dance	to first.
Melpomene:	Muse of Tragedy	
Thalia:	Muse of Comedy	
Polymnia:	Muse of Lyric Tragedy	
Urania:	Muse of Astronomy	
Calliope:	Muse of Eloquence	
Erato:	Muse of Elegy	

It is also possible, according to the intellectual capacity of the pupil, to use the names of various sports, liberal or other professions, cereals, stone fruits, nuts, medicinal herbs, countries, continents, actresses, writers, politicians, poets, etc.

Exercise 3:

Movements of the body.	Lower the body by bending knees. Raise.
Arm movements.	"Squirrel in the cage" exercise, carried out well away from the body.
Speech.	Non-differentiated articulation ("stuttering") should be practised in a whisper on the down movements, and aloud on the rising upright movement (5 minutes per day).

Exercise 4:

Starting position:
Standing, legs together   One arm raised,
        One arm lowered.

Raise and lower each arm in dissociated movements, the one being raised as the other is lowered.

Move one leg backward, then forward; carry on with the two legs alternately.

Move one leg backward, forward, then rest while the other leg carries out the same movement. Enumerate the following types of words, in time with the movements:

Homonym ⎫
Synonym ⎪   Practise this exercise 6 times.
Paronym ⎬
Antonym ⎭

and ask the pupil to provide examples of each, two per division.

EXAMPLES: *faint   feint* ⎫
         sea   see   ⎬ *homonyms*

         hit   strike ⎫
         rapid   swift ⎬ *synonyms*

         crack   track ⎫
         bill   mill ⎬ *paronyms*

         rough   smooth ⎫
         sharp   blunt ⎬ *antonyms*

It can be seen that these exercises can also provide training for the imagination.

Exercise 5:

Hands on the hips, body upright.
Remain completely immobile during the exercise.
Recite by heart or read off a series of sentences with harmoniously balanced stresses.
Eight sentences per session.

Exercise 6: *Same position — complete immobility.*

The pupil is made to repeat a fairly ordinary sentence, suggested by the teacher, with certain given variations of feeling, which are conveyed by suitable types of mimicry.

EXAMPLE: *It is essential to be able to express oneself easily.*

This sentence is repeated so as to convey, by means of intonation and mimicry, the following feelings:

Astonished pleasure–distrust and fear–abusive rage–pained surprise–frank enthusiasm–polite indifference–aggressive indifference–interrogation–resignation–pity–agreement–opposition–entreaty.

Six phrases at each period. Practice in front of a mirror is especially valuable for this exercise.

Exercise 7: In the case of a male or female stammerer whose profession carries certain verbal obligations, each period should include a short impromptu piece on some subject at the time of the exercise. The pupil should be asked to articulate clearly and to speak unhurriedly. Do not thwart him by demanding a slow syllabic utterance, which can result in muscle contractions and provoke further spasms of stammering.

Exercise 8: Reading in a very loud voice. Ask the pupil to imagine that he is reading to a group of people. Two or three pages of text is a suitable length.

Exercise 9: Conversation with the pupil on some subject of particular interest to him, either from the professional point of view, or in relation to his childhood, his family or his academic and religious experience; if relevant his military service may be covered. If the patient is a girl, the discussion may be given a female slant; travel, holidays, family life provide ample material. The field is wide and these conversations should be sufficiently interesting to get the problem of stammering out of the foreground of the patient's mind. In fact it not infrequently happens that a patient loses all sense of proportion with his disability and its psychic consequences. He must as far as possible he helped to escape from this psychosomatic prison. This is the task of the remedial worker, who is his guide, philosopher and friend.

Exercise 10: If it can be achieved, Dr. Chazal has recommended meetings between five or six patients who stammer, in which case the course of the conversation must be skilfully controlled. A subject of collective discussion can be suggested and eventually a sort of colloquium held. The subject of stammering must at all costs be avoided since the object of such colloquia is to make the subjects forget their disability. For this reason the meeting must be run by the teacher.*

* Dr. Chazal. *Le Bégaiement* (Stammering) 1961.

EXERCISES IN THE LYING POSITION
(Psycho-neural motor co-ordination)

Refer for these exercises to the chapter devoted to this type of remedial education for children. All the elements contained in that chapter are suitable for adaptation and for the elaboration of other forms of psycho-neural motor co-ordination exercises.

I cannot reiterate the point too often that multisensory remedial techniques, as applied to psycho-neural motor co-ordination defects, arrhythmic and inhibition disorders which form the serious cases of tonic stammering, *must* be adapted to the individual's psychic, somatic and personality characteristics and to the sufferer's particular state of susceptibility and emotivity.

CHAPTER XII

CREATION OF THE VOX PER OESOPHAGUM IN LARYNGECTOMY PATIENTS

It is of the greatest importance to persuade surgeons of the advantage of creating the vox per oesophagum in their patients prior to the operation. Purely material considerations, such as the difficulty of accommodating the patient in hospital prior to the operation and the complications involved in giving the future patient preventive training, none of which accord with the dictates of common sense, generally result in these patients only being sent to us when the scar has healed sufficiently to allow speech training to be carried out. Pre-operative training is, however, carried out in certain cases. This procedure should have all possible support. A patient whose larynx is still intact is better able to understand and achieve the act of "eructation", on which his speech will subsequently be based. From the physical point of view he is better disposed to receive treatment.

The operative shock and the result of the anaesthetic weaken and depress such patients; they do not appear to possess the necessary powers of application to master the initial gulping stages of the vox per oesophagum. They find themselves in a new and unknown world; this distresses and upsets them and diverts their output of energy. Forewarned is forearmed, and, if they have already produced sounds by "belching" (I must apologise for the use of this rather vulgar term, but it is important to get our meaning over to the patient) the appearance of unexpected compensatory sounds will not come as too great a shock. Otherwise we have to add to their condition of physical debility and distress at losing their larynx the burden of learning an unaccustomed movement.

We should put ourselves in the place of our patients. Only then will we be able to appreciate how much the blow can be softened by teaching them in advance the movements, so difficult for some, which their future condition will require.

REMEDIAL TREATMENT

It goes without saying that the preparatory exercises for the production of the vox per oesophagum require the exercise of great tact and a gentle approach on the part of the remedial worker. The most difficult and the most critical task in the earlier "Education" (and not "Re-education") sessions is to convince the patient that his respiratory apparatus will no longer serve to produce phonetic sounds. One might just as well try to play a violin after removing the strings.

As in all matters affecting human beings the speed at which the first lessons are mastered varies very greatly. Some patients take no time at all; others are slower; some unfortunately never succeed. Age and profession are the governing factors in the creation of this type of phonation. In the case of a young subject and one whose profession requires that he should be able to speak, positive, tangible results can be achieved. With a subject of more mature age, however, or one without a profession, or retired, only great effort and zeal on the part of both teacher and pupil will produce results.

In any case the effort to succeed is the important thing. This is a task requiring passion, tenacity, tact and enthusiasm. On occasion it can be disappointing.

EXERCISES

Exercise 1: Make the patient breathe in and out, stop and belch (belch loudly). He should breathe in, breathe out, swallow and belch. This action, initially so difficult, is soon mastered and becomes automatic; the compensatory adaptation of the organs of the body is of great assistance. In the absence of vocal cords the upper edges of the oesophagus substitute for them. The patient should be made to place his hands on the thoracic edge and feel for himself the sensation of "belching" in the oesophagus.

To assist in the work during the early periods and at home, gas formation for purposes of belching should be promoted by swallowing small gulps of mineral or soda water. The quantities should be kept small and the practice ceased as soon as belching is achieved easily.

Exercise 2: Right from the beginning sound must be transformed into a consonant.

The unvoiced consonants *pe–ke–te* are the easiest; *fe* is harder to obtain initially.

Work should be restricted to what can be achieved with ease; avoid introducing difficulties too early. The patient must be accustomed to the new tonal quality of his "voice". The vox per oesophagum is deeper than the normal voice and tends to sound hoarse. It is none the less beyond dispute that a laryngectomy patient, who is well trained and skilful, can effect a great improvement in the vocal sounds he emits, making them audible and not unpleasant.

Initially *pa–ka–ta* should be practised, followed by *sha* and *fa* (always with the vowel *a*).

Exercise 3: Begin to tackle syllables containing vowels. This is a matter of trial and careful observation.

Have the patient attempt to articulate his best consonant and pronounce it with certain vowels. The unvoiced phoneme *ka*, for example, might be associated with *a–ee–o–oo*, which are all generally easy sounds to produce.

Exercise 4: Proceed with the production of consonants and vowels: *she–zhe–le–fe–ve*. Watch all the time the suspension of the respiration and the belching action.

Explain to the patient that he must take a gulp of air and belch it up immediately. Instruct him to practise the whole day for a certain period in order to make the procedure automatic. This can always be achieved, provided the patient is sufficiently intelligent, zealous and industrious.

Exercise 5 : The consonant *r* is then associated with the syllables, which have already been achieved: *bra–gra–kra–vra–tra–dra.* Attempt the same syllables with different vowels.

EXAMPLES: *bro–kree–gran–cray–troo–droo–froo–vray* etc.

Exercise 6 : Try as far as is possible a few two-syllable words:

EXAMPLES: *copper, batter, parted, coffee, curtain, Paris, pocket, gibbon, rotten, volley, bison, noted, butter, tendon, tappet, tablet, gander, cotter, carter.*

These words cannot be mastered immediately. Those which are articulated best should be studied and repeated *ad nauseam.*

Never insist on the patient struggling with a word which is badly pronounced. At all costs he must not be allowed to become discouraged, tired and tense. Watch carefully that he is not producing the sounds during inspiration, which could be dangerous. The teacher must be constantly on the alert and attentive.

Exercise 7 : The consonant *l*, the sibilants and the nasals *m* and *n* take a fairly long time to obtain. They should be studied initially within the framework of words:

EXAMPLES: *ally, olive, emit, Anna, pony, pommel, allay, assist, pussy, poser, razor, assent, palace, howler, paling, Polly.*

I have given above a brief review of how the remedial treatment should be tackled. There are many possible variants since we have to be quite indefatigable in adapting methods and techniques to the daily needs of our patients... Never try to go too fast. Make sure that what is learnt is learnt properly and for good.

Exercise 8: Get the patient accustomed to producing words of three or four syllables in one belch. Never divide up words between belches. This is too difficult.

Practise short phrases to start with.

EXAMPLE: "I drink coffee" not "I ... drink ... coff ...ee".

It is a good thing to conjugate these short phrases throughout one tense of the verb.

EXAMPLES: "I read the letter, You read the letter" etc. Describe the course of your day. "I get up at such and such a time. I wash or I take a bath. I have my breakfast. I shave. I read the paper or listen to the news", and so on throughout the day.

Exercise 9:

When progress has been made with the treatment, start reading aloud. In dealing with educated patients, use can be made of the stress, to practise the rhythmic balance of the belched sounds.

The patient may also be made to recount a fable or recite a poem or practise calling or answering on the telephone.

EXAMPLE: "Hallo, this is John Smith speaking". The slight emotional response involved in answering the telephone provides an excellent opportunity for a handicapped subject to exercise his skill in the spoken language. The patient must be urged to try this, although every effort must be made to avoid upsetting or putting too great a strain on him.

Exercise 10: The results achieved are sometimes encouraging. It is a good thing, when the patient has begun to express himself with a fair degree of fluency, to ask him to give a short talk on some subject which can then be recorded on the tape recorder. This can be a great stimulus, both to the patient, his family and to the teacher as well.

It is clear, and one must have the courage to say so, that the success achieved by this form of phoniatric treatment is often not in proportion to the trouble taken or the efforts made. Right from the start of the remedial sessions the possibilities of achieving phonetic and vocal success can be foreseen. The patient either understands and carries out the instructions ... or not.

If all is well, things can go quite fast. One may hope to create an acceptable voice in a few weeks, six or eight for example. The laryngectomy patient should also be given articulation exercises (maxilla, lips, tongue) which cannot but help to promote the acquisition of speech. We must, however, expect setbacks and complications for reasons over which we have no control. Sometimes the tracheal orifice is blocked with mucous matter, which impedes the patient. The tracheal "cannula" often requires to be replaced or modified; the patient coughs, which impedes the work on phonation and articulation, and he also may suffer gastric pain. There are finally various hazards which may impede or compromise the effect of remedial treatment.

All possible irritating and aggravating circumstances have to be endured but one should never lose patience or hope. Success, when achieved, is the finest possible reward for the efforts we have made. The results are sometimes quite decisive. One laryngectomy patient was able recently, after two months of treatment, to make a short address in public (at a meeting of a trade union, of which the patient was president). Another has been able to resume his occupation as a commercial representative. Such conclusive successes are not always achieved. I must emphasize the fact (the consequences of which are only too apparent) that laryngectomy patients are frequently the victims of anxiety, obsession and hyperemotionality. I have found it an excellent practice to hold relaxation periods on the analogy of those held for dysphonic patients; these have a calming influence on the vegetative nervous system and both for the reduction of mucous matter and coughs I have been able to record clear improvements in this way.

Research is at present being carried out to facilitate the recovery of the voice in laryngectomy patients. I do not know whether the aids at present available are easy to use and of benefit to the user. I sincerely hope that some improvement may be made in this way in the phonetic capacity of such patients. In any case the training of the vox per oesophagum, the substitute voice, still represents the best available hope for the future of the laryngectomy patient in his family and in society. He may well achieve normal speech. This depends also on the operative technique applied and the extent of the intervention. If the surgeon has left intact certain of the muscles and of the branches of the oesophagal nerves and the recurrent nerves, we have here a precious foundation on which to build the vox per oesophagum. In this case, however, as in many others, every one does what he is able and adapts himself to the amount of damage that has been done and to the dangers that exist.

A NOTE ON DEAFNESS IN ADULTS

I shall only devote a few lines to cases of deafness in adults. This is above all the sphere of the doctor. The advances which have taken place over the years in surgery and medicine, and the vast improvement in hearing aids have greatly lightened the burden of patients with defective hearing. In principle, at least, their lives have become tolerable and for some the combination of surgery and the hearing aid have restored them to normal life.

Remedial education is of use in connection with the hearing aid, in order to re-establish and train auditory habits and to mitigate the difficulties resulting from a disparity between the bilateral auditory fields. Those who are fitted with hearing aids, however, tend to fall into two classes: those whose hearing is so much improved that they need no assistance, and those who entrench themselves behind the barrier of their infirmity and, quite disillusioned, abandon all attempts to overcome it, including remedial treatment. It is the task of the orthophonist* to provide instruction in lip-reading and training in normal articulation, an aspect of the training of the deaf which I have often found to be most neglected. The deaf subject, even if he is made to hear almost normally, must attempt to improve his speech and language so as to be able to understand and make himself understood.

* In Britain this work is undertaken by qualified teachers of the deaf.

The deaf person who has not received proper care or whose condition is not amenable to treatment, is one of life's failures. If he does not possess unusual spiritual stamina he will give way under the weight of his physical distress and the blow to his morale. We might quote as an example the greatest genius of them all, the immortal Beethoven, who by superhuman effort produced his "Hymn of Joy" at the moment when, overwhelmed with bitterness and disappointment, he was ending the life which had been one long martyrdom. It was in 1796, when he was 26, that the first symptoms of deafness developed and sorrow took its place at his fireside. The sound of moaning and groaning was present in his ears night and day and he became an exile in his own world. All he could hear were the melodies that rang deep within him. It was in this dark night of deafness that Beethoven composed his *Ninth Symphony*, his *Mass in D*, the last five sonatas and the last six quartets.

Today life has changed for the deaf person. Highly effective surgical intervention has eliminated or considerably reduced the suffering of some categories of deaf subjects. Hearing aids also have contributed greatly to easing the burden, which these unfortunates have to bear. Remedial teachers can still be of assistance to the serious, incurable cases of deafness, where surgical intervention of any sort is not effective. We can still help these serious cases by a combination of lip-reading and phonetic exercises. It is, however, rare for these unfortunates to conform to the discipline of remedial education. The treatment is long, the patient becomes tired and very often he gives up after a relatively short period. Lip-reading techniques are, moreover, too well and too widely known for me to spend time describing them.

4735

Made in Great Britain